our remarkable feet

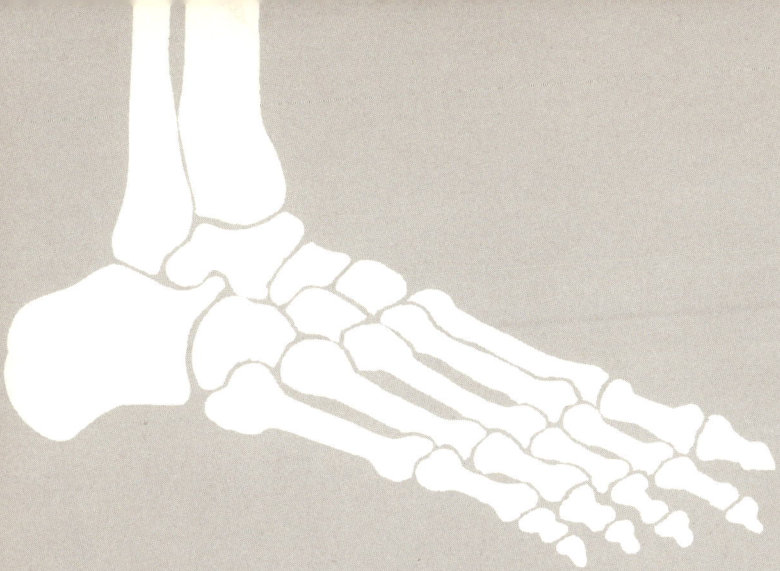

our remarkable feet

By
Robert K. Krishef
Illustrated by
Harold K. Lamson

Published by
Lerner Publications Company
Minneapolis, Minnesota

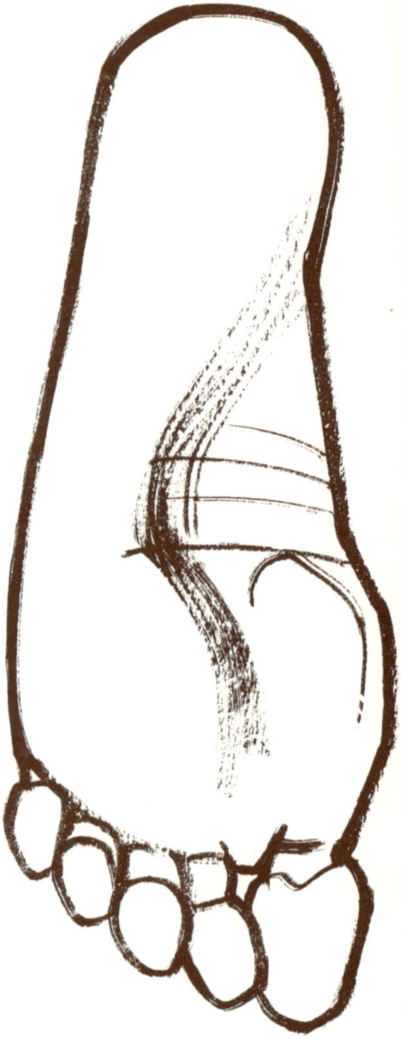

Library of Congress Number: 67-30693

Second Printing 1968

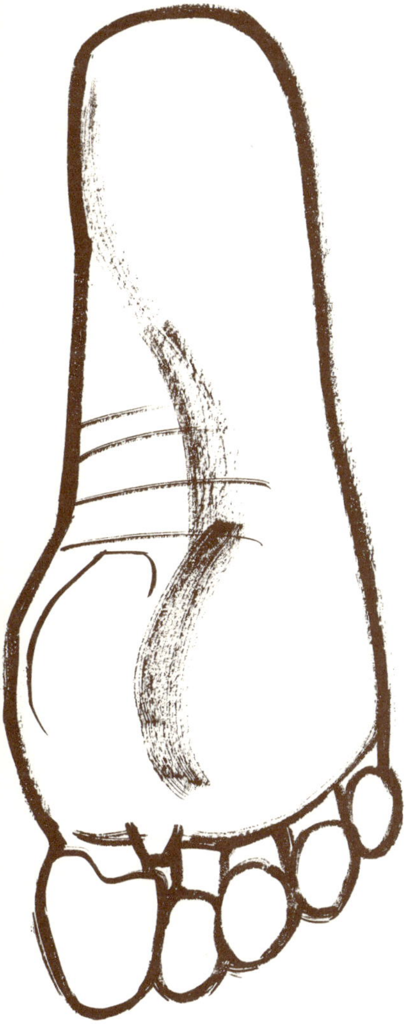

contents

Introduction 7
Chapter I
Structure of the Foot 8
Chapter II
How We Move 12
Chapter III
The Foot At Work 17
Chapter IV
Walking for Pleasure 22
Chapter V
Games, Fun and Ceremony 25
Chapter VI
Aids and Accessories 32
Chapter VII
The Study of the Feet 39
Conclusion
The Future of the Foot 44

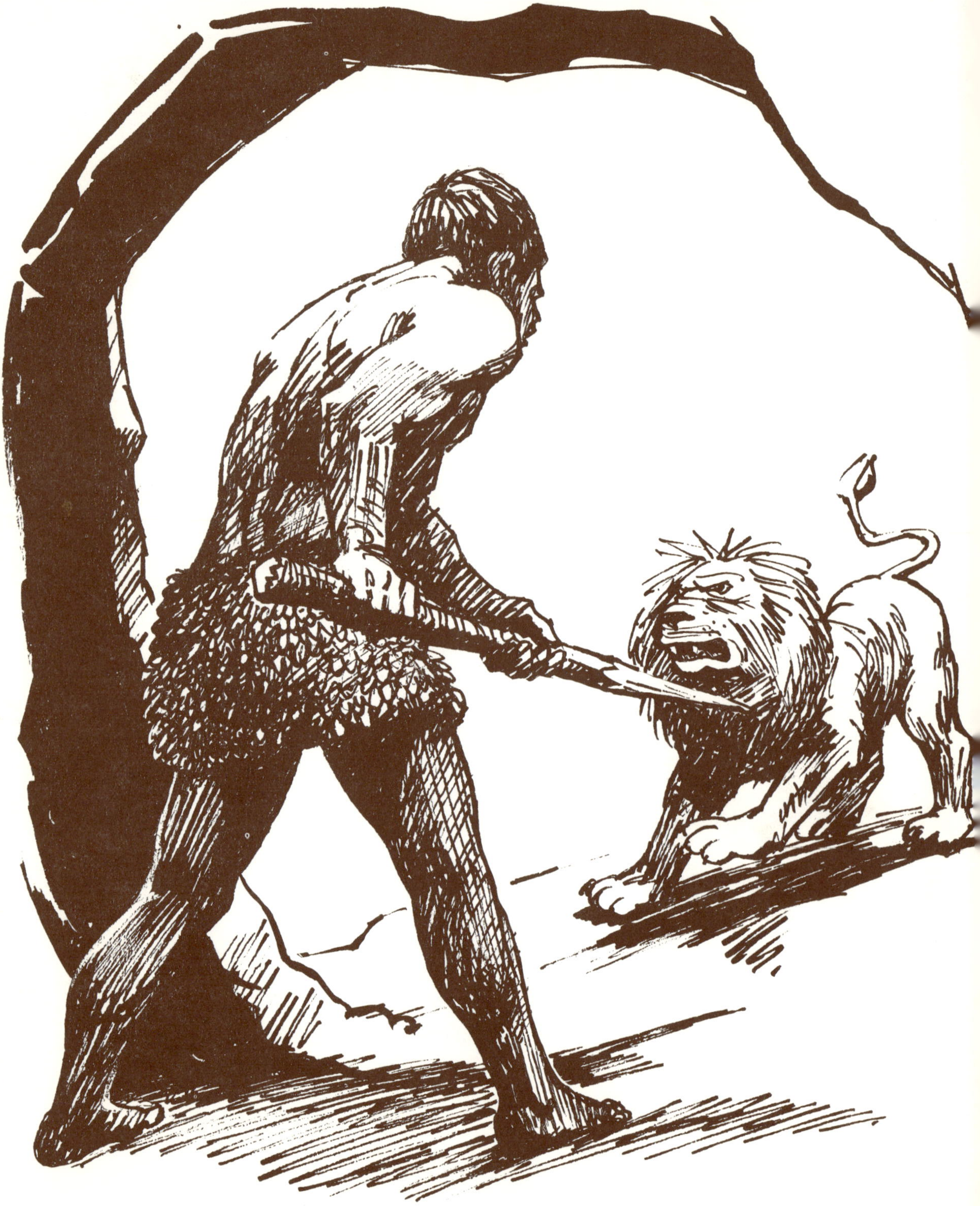

introduction

Long, long ago man and the animal kingdom fought for superiority. It appeared to be an uneven battle, because man in many ways seemed very puny compared to his foe.

Some animals were far stronger than human beings. Some animals were much faster. Some were stronger *and* faster.

In other respects, too, man was at a disadvantage. He did not have sharp claws for climbing trees. He did not have sharp teeth to use against his enemies. He did not have such keen senses of smell and hearing as did many animals.

How, then, did our primitive ancestors become dominant? The answer, of course, is that the human body has amazing abilities of its own. With our brain, we can think and plan. With our power of speech, we can teach, work with others, and pass on knowledge from one generation to another. With our hands, we can grasp objects and make things.

Gradually, man developed these skills. He learned to use them together, and this teamwork within the body was vital. For example, because he could stand and walk erect, on his two feet, man's hand was free to become a valuable tool. Without this tool, he undoubtedly would not have survived.

Walking, of course, is not ordinarily considered a skill. Neither is our ability to talk, to hold a hammer, and to perform hundreds of apparently simple tasks. Yet, have you ever watched a baby walk for the first time, or listened to him try to talk?

We are not born with skills, but we are born with the ability to *acquire* them. They become simple only after we have repeated them so often that we no longer really think about what we are doing. It is automatic, or subconscious — but no less wonderful.

There are many intricate and remarkable parts to the human body. One of those parts is the foot, which particularly suits the needs of man. We have depended upon it and it has served us well, from the very beginning of civilization.

Chapter I THE STRUCTURE OF THE FOOT

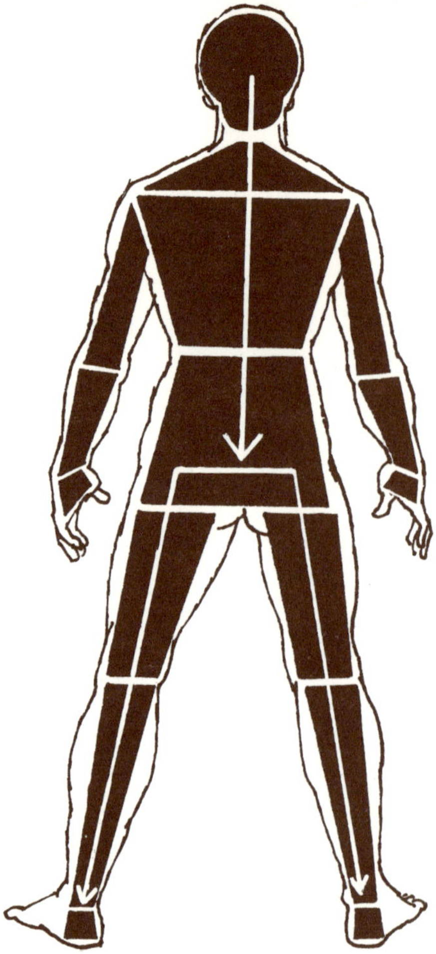

Footings are the bottom support of a building or a bridge. In their planning, the builder and architect must be certain that the footings are firm and strong enough to hold the weight of the building or bridge. Otherwise, the structure eventually would topple.

This has given us expressions or phrases which we use in other ways. We speak of an idea as needing a "firm foundation." A successful businessman is particularly proud if he worked his way "from the bottom up." In talking about the body, we also could well begin at the bottom—with the strength and firm foundation provided by the feet.

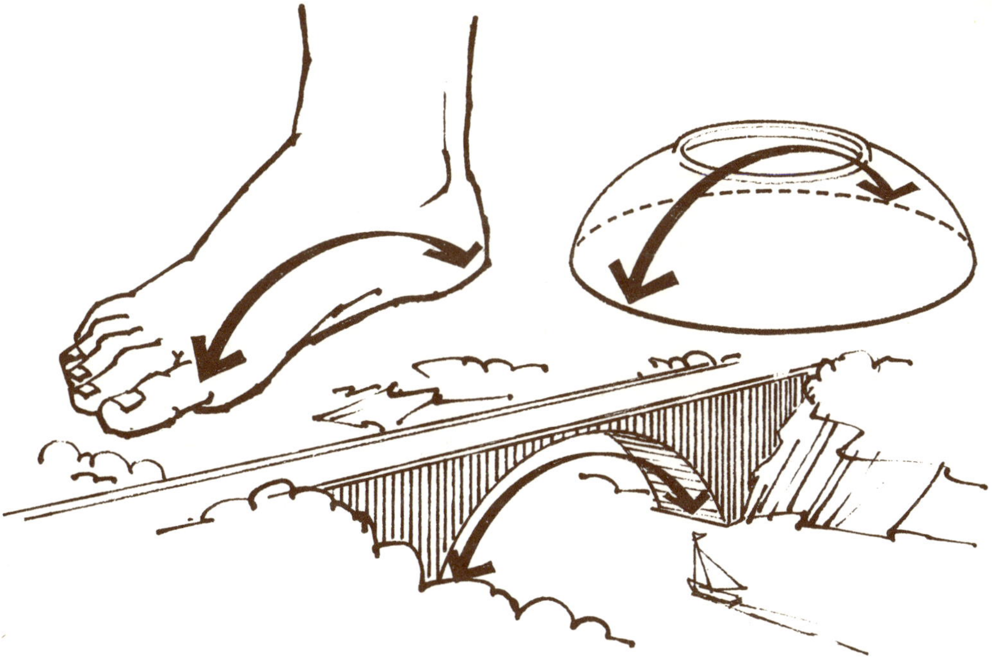

The feet support the body

When we stand, the feet support the weight of the entire body, just as footings support the weight of the building. Furthermore, to measure strain on the feet during walking, we must add the weight of the body with each step taken. When you simply walk around the block, without carrying anything, the number of pounds absorbed by your feet is far greater than the weight of a family automobile.

Normally, however—and fortunately, too—we are not aware of this pressure. The reason is that the foot is constructed in a very special way. It has an arch, which means that the bones fit with one another so that part of the foot is raised slightly. This construction, curving like a shallow upside-down bowl, relieves the foot of pressure without weakening it.

The same principle has often been used in the construction of bridges—from little foot-overpasses to bridges the length of several city blocks. If you look beneath an arched bridge, you will see how its supports are curved. The first person to successfully build such a bridge may have gotten his idea from the human foot.

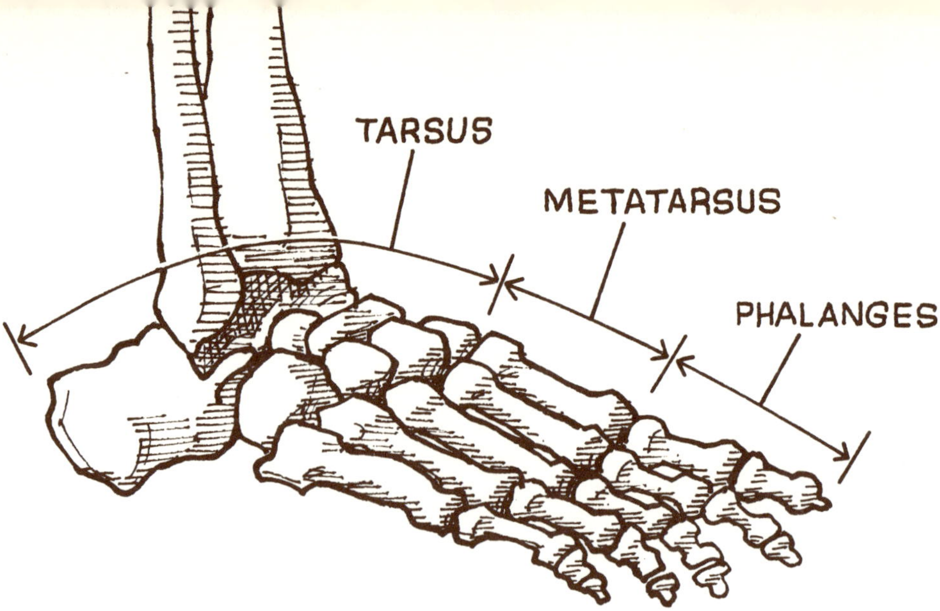

Structure of the foot

It takes an unusually large number of parts to form an arch in the foot. Each foot has 26 bones. Combined, the feet have about one-fourth of the bones in the entire human body, which altogether has 206 bones.

The bones of the foot are divided into three groups: the *tarsus,* the *metatarsus,* and the *phalanges.*

The tarsus comprises the back part of the foot. It includes the ankle bone and heel bone, plus five chunky bones in front of them.

Meta is a word meaning "beyond" or "between." The metatarsus is the middle part of the foot, beyond the tarsus or between the tarsus and phalanges. There are five straight, narrow bones in this group. The foot is held up in an arch because of the firmly constructed vertical curve made by the tarsus and metatarsus, and the equally strong horizontal curve made by the metatarsus.

The underpart of the metatarsal region of the foot is called the sole. The upper part is the instep. The heads of the five metatarsal bones form the ball of the foot. Each head is connected to one of the five phalanges, which are the toes. There are two bones in the big toe, and three in each of the other toes.

The strongest bone in the foot is the heel. It has to be, because it strikes the ground first when we walk. For an instant, it is supporting all of the body weight, which has been passed to it from the ankle bone. As the rest of the foot hits the ground, the pressure is distributed to several of the other bones, going from one bone to another like an object passing from hand to hand. The destination of this pressure is the big

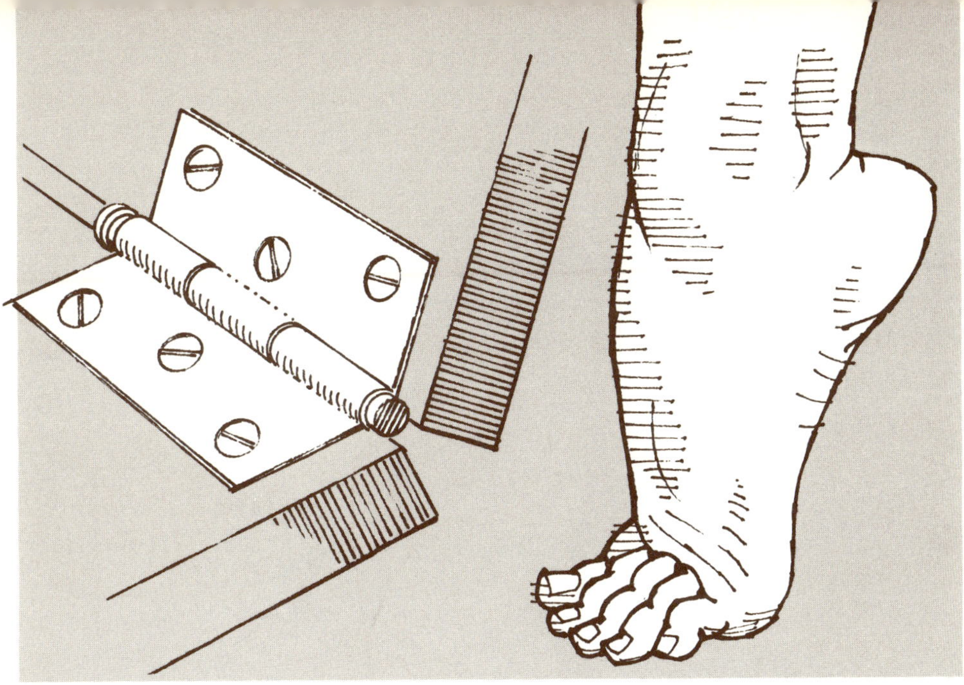

toe. This toe, with some help from the other toes, then pushes the body forward.

Flexibility

Our feet are designed for graceful walking. The toes are quite flexible, as you can see when you wiggle or bend them. Some people who have lost the use of their hands have even learned to write or paint by holding the pencil or brush between their toes. The foot itself is also extremely versatile. It can be moved at the ankle from side to side, and up and down. If you have ever had an injured ankle or a sore toe, you know how this affects the use of the foot.

The flexibility of our feet, like the movements of other parts of the body, is possible because of the way the bones are attached. Bones are tied together with bands of elastic material called *ligaments.* At the point of connection there is a joint, which is a special arrangement of the bones, like a door hinge. This special arrangement allows movement, and also includes a layer of *cartilage* or padding, to prevent the bones from scraping.

Within the cartilage is a pliable lining that discharges fluid. The fluid keeps the joint lubricated so that it works smoothly, just as lubricating oil keeps a machine working smoothly.

Of course a machine needs more than lubrication. It must be started, and operated properly. The same is true of the human body. Let's see next how our feet "get moving."

Chapter II HOW WE MOVE

There is a football story about a halfback who boasted about his long gains. His teammates decided to teach him a lesson the next time he carried the ball. They did not block the opposing players for him. Of course the halfback was tackled for a loss, which made him realize how important teamwork was.

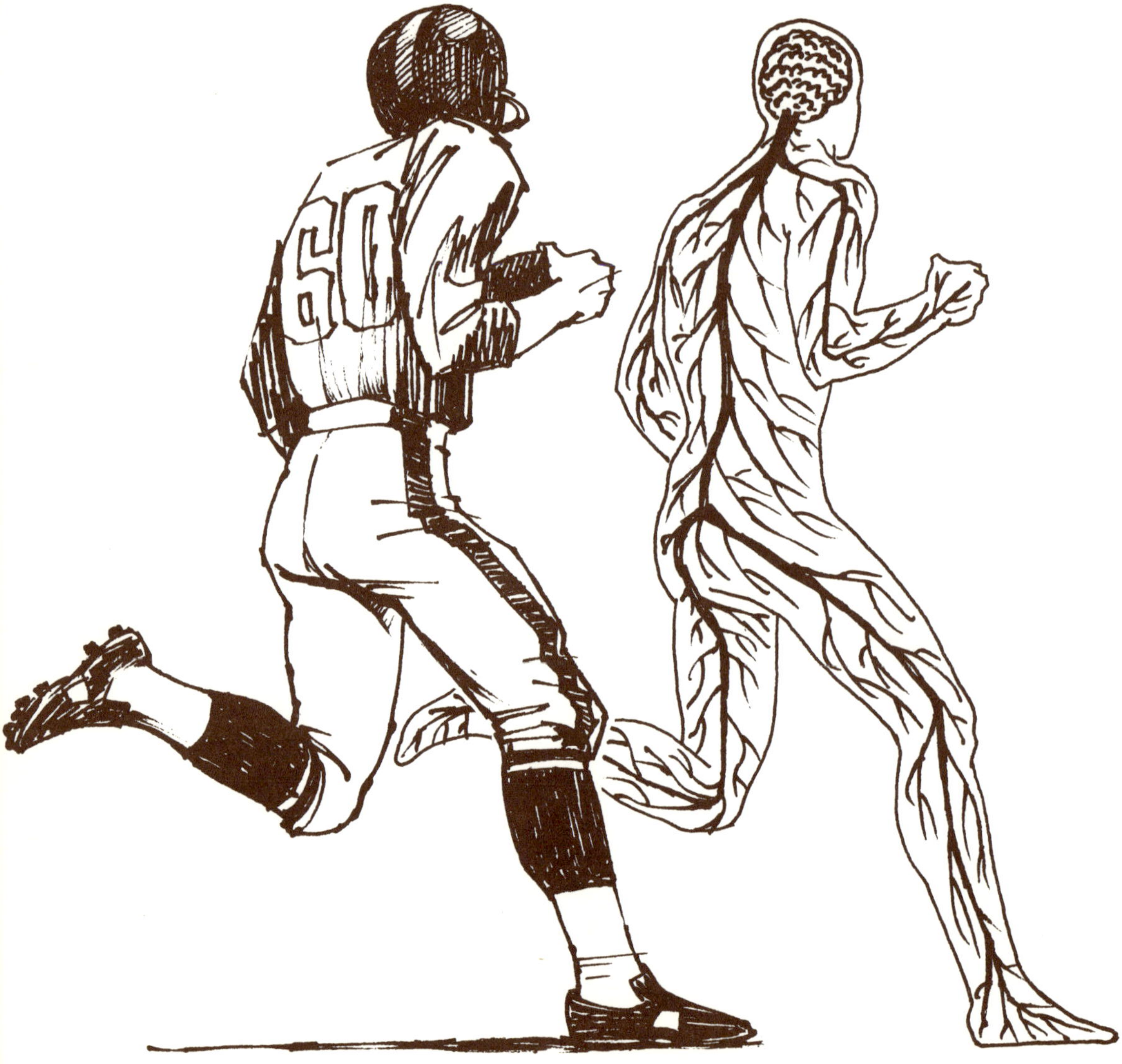

Teamwork is required within the human body, too. Our feet are remarkably constructed, with bones that are very strong and durable. But they need help from other parts of the body, just as the halfback needed help from other members of the team.

In football, the quarterback calls the plays and the signals. He decides who will carry the ball, and in what direction. In the body, the brain is the quarterback. It sends orders or signals which cause us to move. When we walk or run, each step is ordered individually by the brain. This happens so quickly, however, that we are not aware of it.

The nervous system

The brain is organized into compartments or sections. The main section is across the upper portion of the head, and is called the *cerebrum.* This is the part of the brain where thoughts are stored and decisions are made. In the back of the head, at the "stem" of the brain, is a part shaped something like a ball. This area is named the *cerebellum,* which is sometimes referred to as the "little brain." It controls body coordination and movement, including movements of the feet. A person cannot walk a straight line or catch a ball properly if his cerebellum has been damaged.

The stem of the brain is connected to the spinal cord, which is in the back of the human body. The spinal cord carries signals from the brain and delivers messages to the brain. These signals and messages leave and enter the spinal cord through a system of nerves and nerve fibers. The fibers spread out from the nerves like branches from a tree. The spinal cord, nerves, and nerve fibers, along with the brain as headquarters, form the body's vast communication network. This network is called the nervous system.

There are two kinds of nerves. Those transmitting signals *from* the brain are *motor nerves.* Through them, the brain directs the body to act or move. Other nerves have receptors, resembling tiny buds, on the tips of their fiber branches. These nerves are *sensory nerves.* Their receptors collect information and sensations which are sent *to* the brain. They tell us whether something is hot or cold, smooth or rough, hard or soft.

We often use both kinds of nerves at almost the same moment. At the beach during the summer, you take off your shoes and socks and step barefoot from a blanket or grass onto the hot sand. Instantly your sensory nerves flash that "ouch" feeling. You react through your motor nerves either by hopping from one foot to the other or by racing for the water!

The muscles

The force or energy for these movements, and for all body activity, is provided by muscles. Muscles consist of bundles of hair-like fibers which are very strong and packed very tightly. These bundles are attached to tough ropes of material called *tendons,* which in turn are attached to the bones. The muscles react to signals from the brain. This reaction moves the tendons, which move the bones.

Two important muscles used by the feet are located in the calf, the part of the leg extending from the knee to the ankle. The strongest and thickest tendon in the body connects those muscles with the heel bone. Hold your calf and flex your foot as though standing on tiptoe, relax, and flex it again. Your brain has sent this order through the spinal cord, and you can feel the muscles and tendon react to the order.

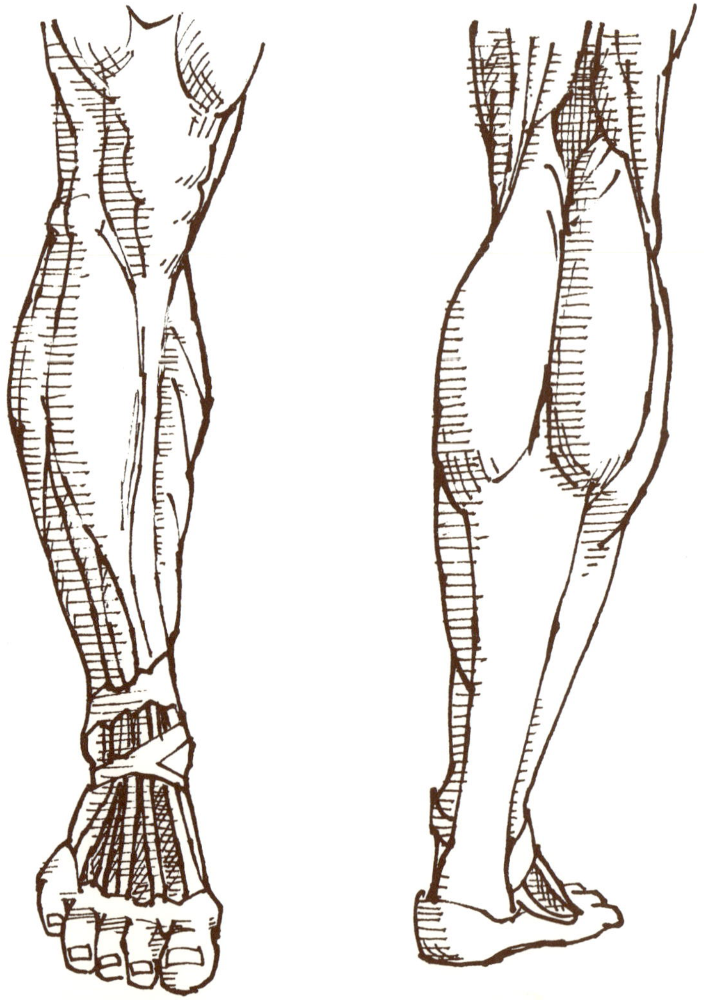

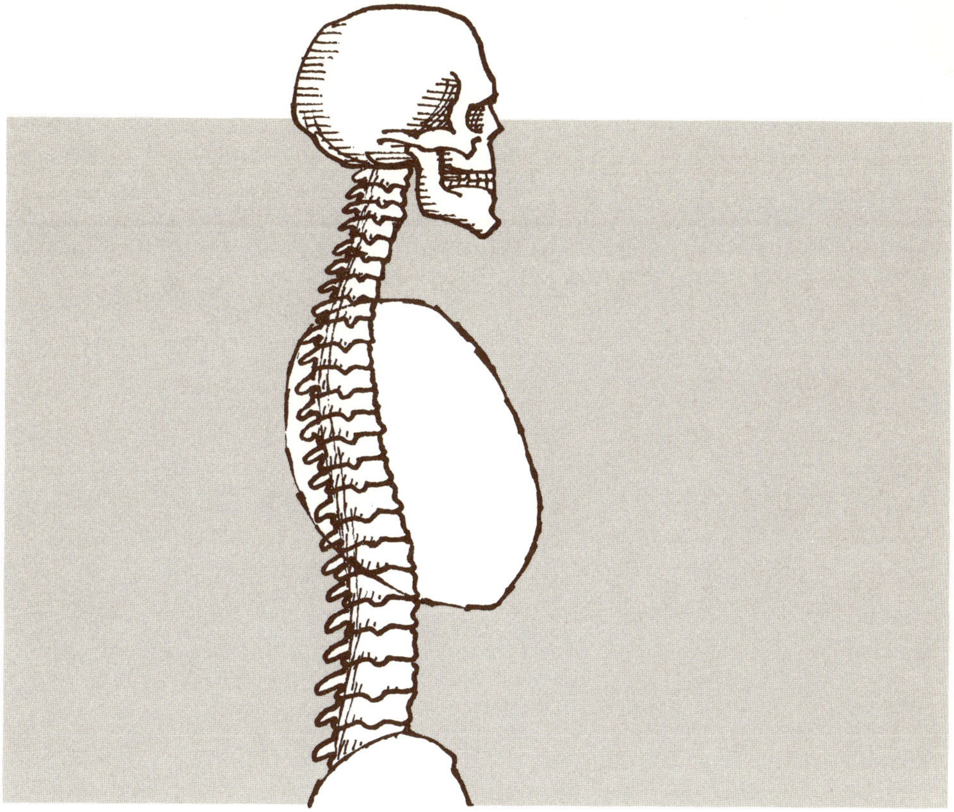

The backbone

The spinal cord is involved in all messages to and from the brain. Fortunately, it is well protected by the spinal column or backbone, which runs down the center of the back.

The backbone is not a single bone. It is a connecting column of 26 individual, doughnut-shaped bones, called vertebrae. The spinal cord passes through the middle of each vertebra like thread through a needle, and is surrounded as though by circles of bodyguards. In addition, bumps and shock are absorbed by spongy cartilage between the vertebrae. Cartilage also makes the backbone flexible, so that we can bend, reach, and stretch.

The backbone is sturdy as well as flexible. We stand on our feet. But we can stand *up* because the backbone can be pulled as rigid as a pole. No other creature is able to stand as comfortably erect as man. This had led to the expression, "He has a lot of backbone," which is an admiring way of describing someone with will-power and character.

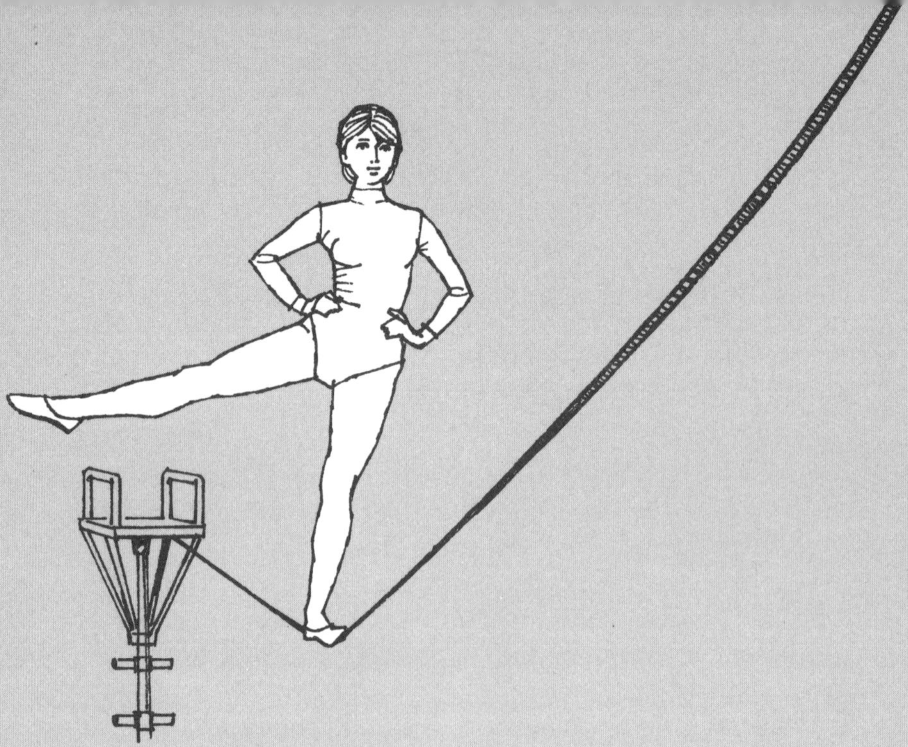

Coordination and balance

Although standing and walking seem simple enough, even these actions require fine coordination. In climbing stairs, for instance, approximately 300 muscles are used. This muscle work must be coordinated with eyesight, with the foot's sense of feeling, and with the body's sense of balance.

The sense of balance actually is part of our hearing apparatus. This apparatus includes an inner ear, which—as the name indicates—is located within the head. The inner ear sends sound messages to the brain. It also has an extremely sensitive system for signaling the brain about the position of the head and body.

In the inner ear are semi-circular canals, filled with fluid and containing special bristles or hairs. Any movement of the head or body shakes or tips the fluid. This stimulates the hairs, alerting the brain as to the direction of the movement. The brain then sends orders to the muscles needed to keep the body in balance.

Some people, such as circus tightrope walkers, develop an especially keen sense of balance and muscle reaction. The rest of us are not trained or skillful enough to perform such daring feats. We are content to use our feet for the normal purposes.

Chapter III THE FOOT AT WORK

Early man used his feet for the same purposes as we do today—to stand, to walk, to run. There is, however, one difference. Those who lived long ago used their feet much more than we do, because walking was their only means of transportation.

An average person today might walk 15,000 to 20,000 steps a day. But the average early man must have taken many more steps than that, in search of food or a better place to make his home. Trying to imagine the number of steps he took during his lifetime is like trying to accurately count the stars in the sky, or grains of sand on a beach. You can get dizzy just thinking about it!

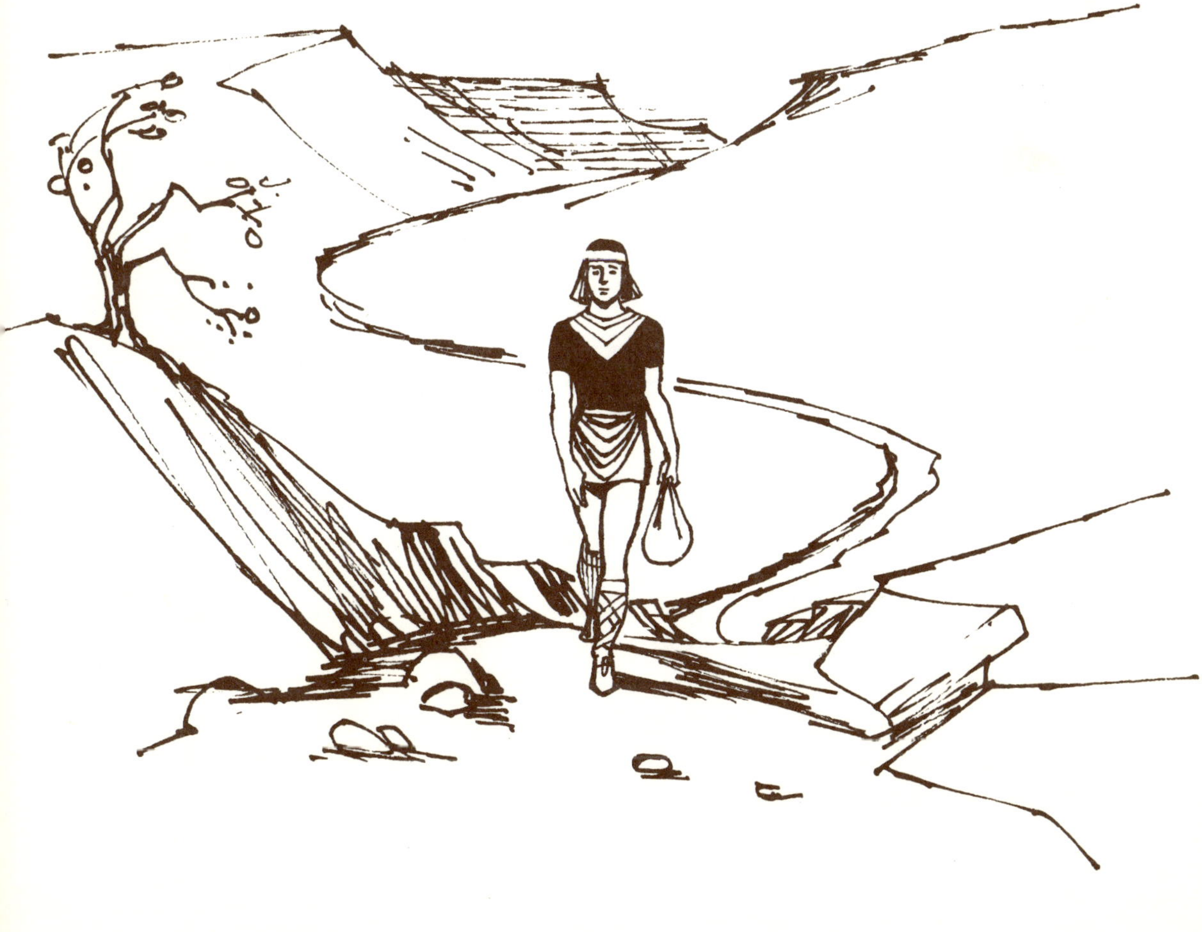

Paths, roads, and highways

Although we cannot know precisely how much man walked, we can be certain of the value of the foot. Many of our modern streets and highways, for instance, follow the original narrow paths pounded out by the footsteps of man through forests, along streams, over hills, and into valleys.

At first, these paths were wide enough for only one person. Gradually, they were enlarged by constant use, as well as by cutting and smashing of grass and tree branches on both sides. With the introduction of the wheel—one of man's greatest inventions—carts and wagons trampled paths into trails. Eventually trails became dusty roads and, finally, surveyors used these same routes to determine where paved streets and highways should go.

History includes many stories of man on foot. Moses and the Hebrews walked for 40 years, seeking their Promised Land of Israel. Jesus, and later His disciples, walked through the countryside as they spread the gospel of Christianity. Some of the disciples probably strolled along roads which had been constructed before the time of Christ by the Roman Empire for its horsemen, chariots, carts, and foot soldiers. Many of the roads had special raised areas in the middle or off to the side for pedestrians, a word meaning "going on foot." These areas were the first known sidewalks.

Our own country was built because the human foot was strong enough to carry men through the wilderness. Some of our famous pioneer roads, such as the Santa Fe Trail to the Southwest, and the Oregon Trail to the Pacific Northwest, were at first paths made by hunters on foot. One of the most famous American trailblazers was Daniel Boone. In 1775, he cut a trail from Virginia through the Appalachian Mountains into Kentucky. This trail was called the Wilderness Road. It was the first path over which pioneers from the 13 colonies could ride or walk into new frontiers.

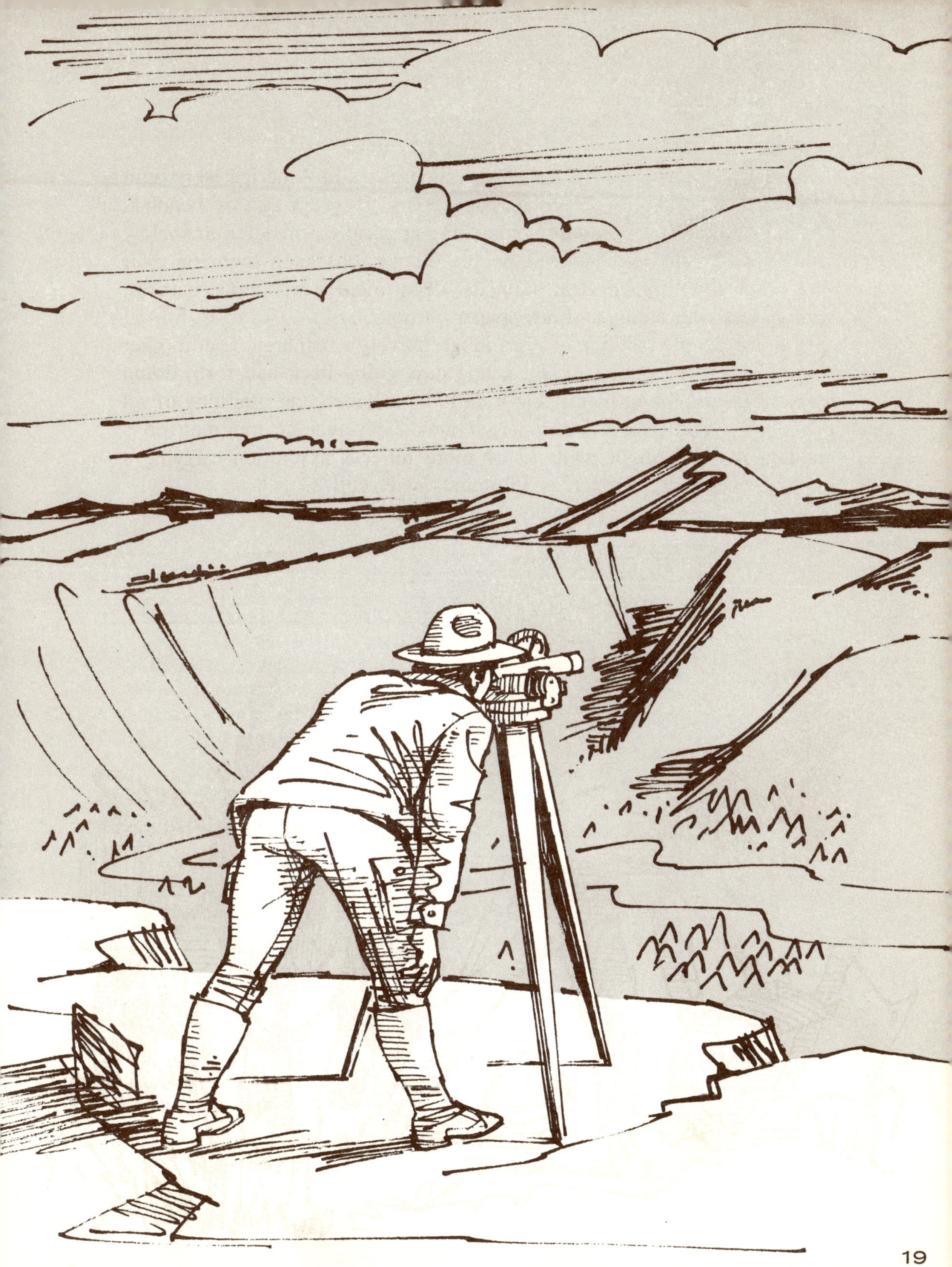

The foot at work

Many of the great industries and businesses in America were built "on foot." They were started perhaps 50 or 75 years ago by peddlers pushing fruit carts, or by junkmen picking up scraps of metal. Our society continues to have and to need people whose jobs keep them on their feet—policemen on the beat, dentists, department store clerks, barbers, waiters and waitresses, and newspaper carrier boys.

Some people take many steps in a relatively small area. Your mother may walk eight or nine miles in one day, going back and forth doing housework and fixing meals. Door-to-door salesmen and mailmen travel even more, and over a much larger area. The average mailman on a residential route might walk 12 or more miles a day, often carrying a mail bag weighing as much as 35 pounds when full.

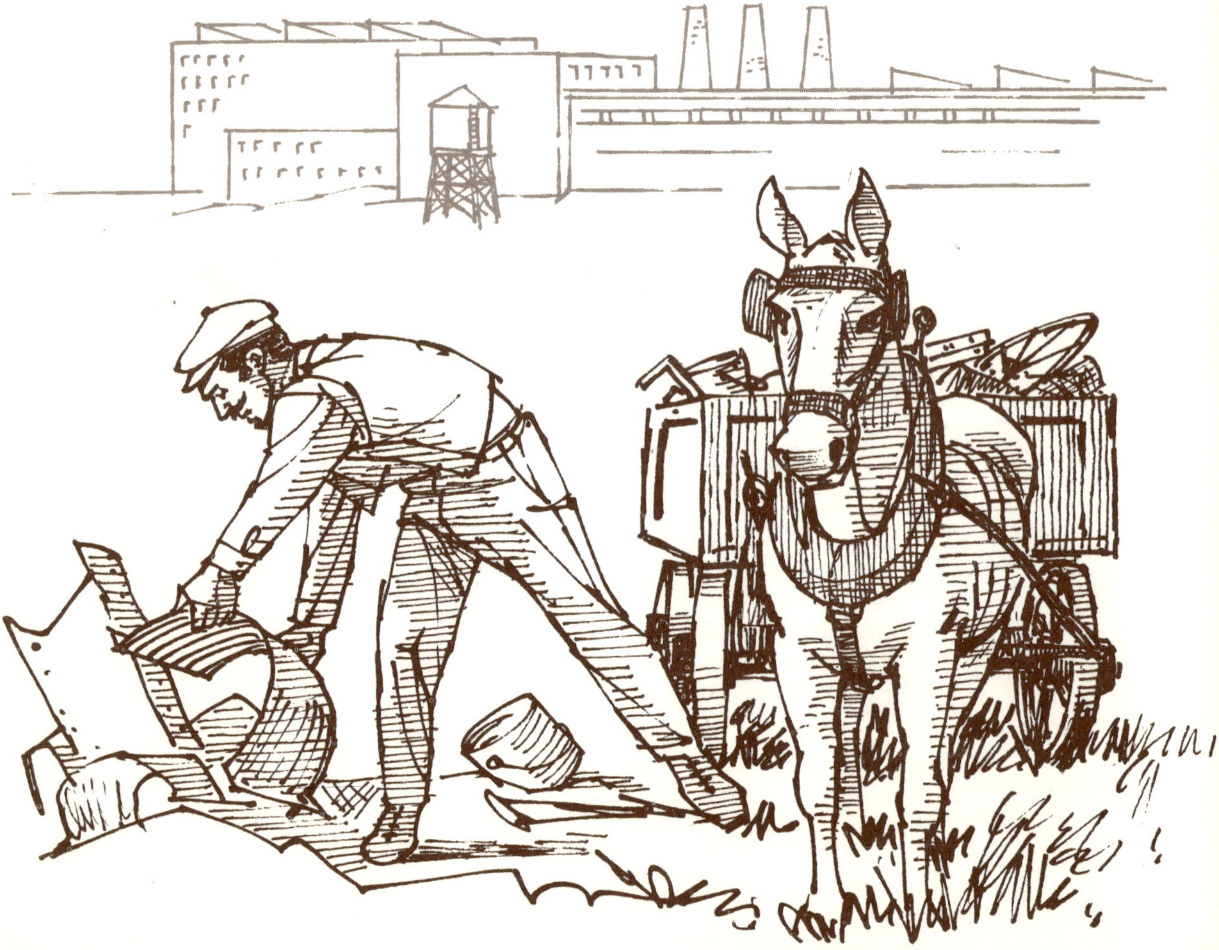

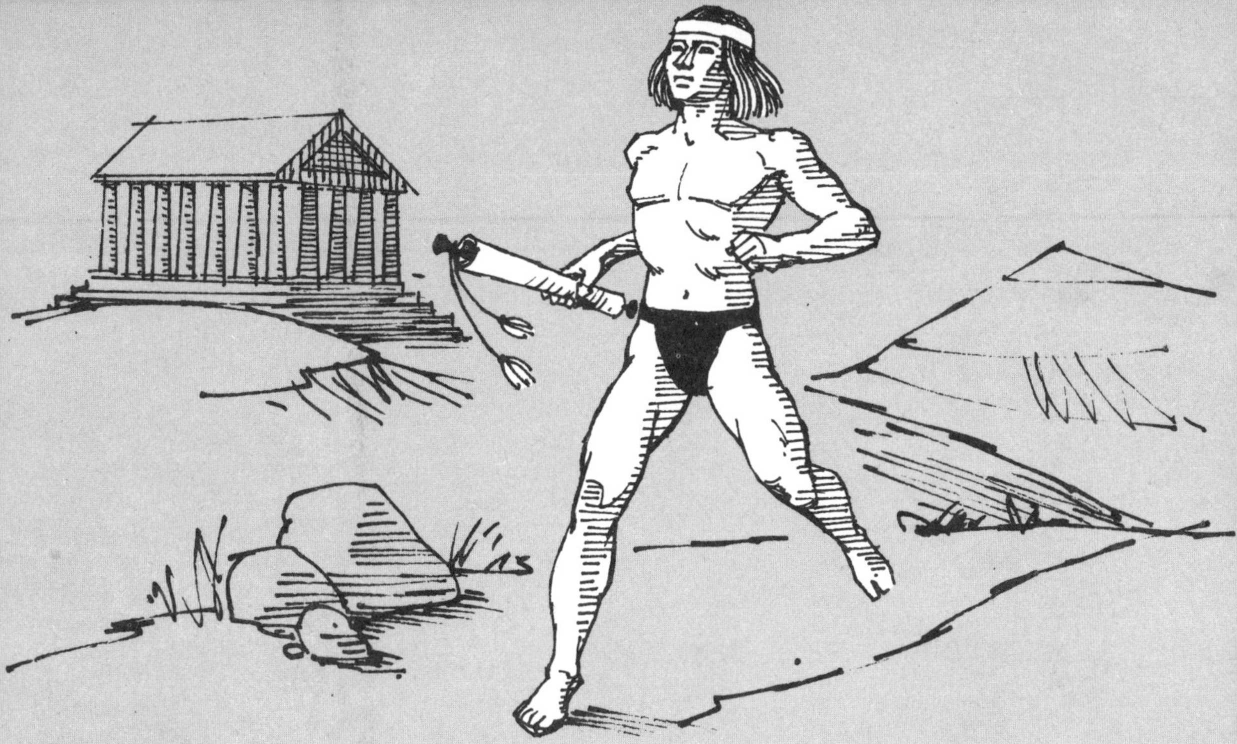

Messengers

The job of delivering mail or messages is a very old one. It must have begun almost immediately after human beings organized into communities and villages. When one village chief wanted to communicate secretly with another, he sent a messenger who was trained to run long distances. This was before man rode horseback.

Even after villages grew into nations, kings depended on the powerful legs and feet of their runners or messengers. Sometimes the runner carried a ring or another token to prove that he was delivering a message from the king.

As new nations formed and expanded, the distances between them were often too great for one runner. So relay stations were put along delivery routes. Fresh messengers took the mail from tired messengers just as, centuries later, our American pony express riders changed horses in carrying mail across the country.

Greece was one of the many nations which, in ancient times, used foot messengers. Their messengers were so respected that these words were written about them: "Neither snow nor rain nor heat nor gloom of night stays these couriers from the swift completion of their appointed rounds." This today is the slogan of our United States Post Office.

Chapter IV WALKING FOR PLEASURE

Some people have jobs which keep them on their feet. Others do not. But away from work, all of us can benefit from the fact that the human foot is built for walking. Should we walk, in this age of the automobile? The answer is "yes." There are three good reasons for taking a walk: Enjoyment. Education. Exercise.

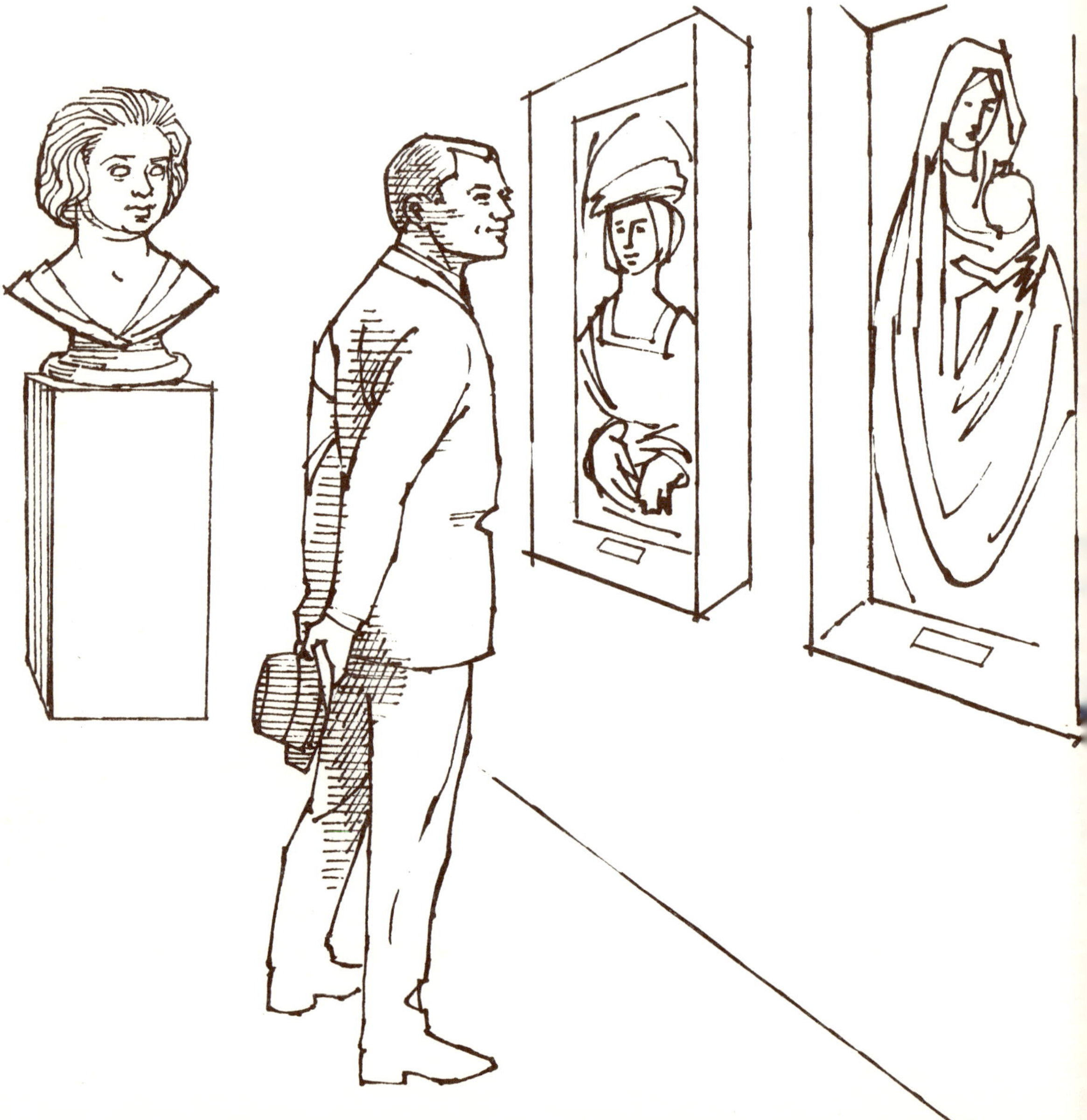

Enjoyment

If one were asked to describe the typical walker, he could not do it accurately. That is because there is no such person. Walking is a hobby which appeals to many different kinds of people, and it is a hobby which is practiced in many different ways.

Walkers come in all shapes and sizes—heavy or thin, tall or short. They walk fast. They walk slow. Some follow the same route every time. Others stroll aimlessly. One person might go for a walk every night at precisely the same hour, for the same number of minutes. Another goes out only when he is in the mood, and walks as long as the mood lasts.

You will find walkers in the rain and under the blazing sun, in the middle of summer or the coldest part of winter. They have in common their enjoyment of walking. But they might explain this enjoyment in different ways —"It relaxes me so I can sleep better," or "It helps me think," or "It makes me feel good and refreshed."

Education

Walking can be educational as well as enjoyable. Many people enjoy walking *because* it is educational. A person on foot has the opportunity to stop, look, and listen. He will know more about nature, history, and people than one who always rides.

Some walkers belong to organized hiking and walking clubs. These clubs have helped other volunteer groups, government officials, and interested individuals in constructing many fine hiking trails throughout the country. The trails or foot-paths are for anyone who wants to use them. These trails pass through national forests and parks, state parks, mountains, and privately owned land. One of the most famous is the Appalachian Trail, which stretches more than 2,000 miles through 13 states in the southeastern and eastern section of the United States.

Much can be learned on foot in the city, too. The best way to explore the many neighborhoods in New York City is on foot. One of New York's museums conducts walking tours of old buildings threatened with demolishment. A museum in Philadelphia sponsors a "Liberty Walk" which includes historic attractions like Independence Hall. Palisades Park in Santa Monica, California and Golden Gate Park in San Francisco attract many visitors on foot.

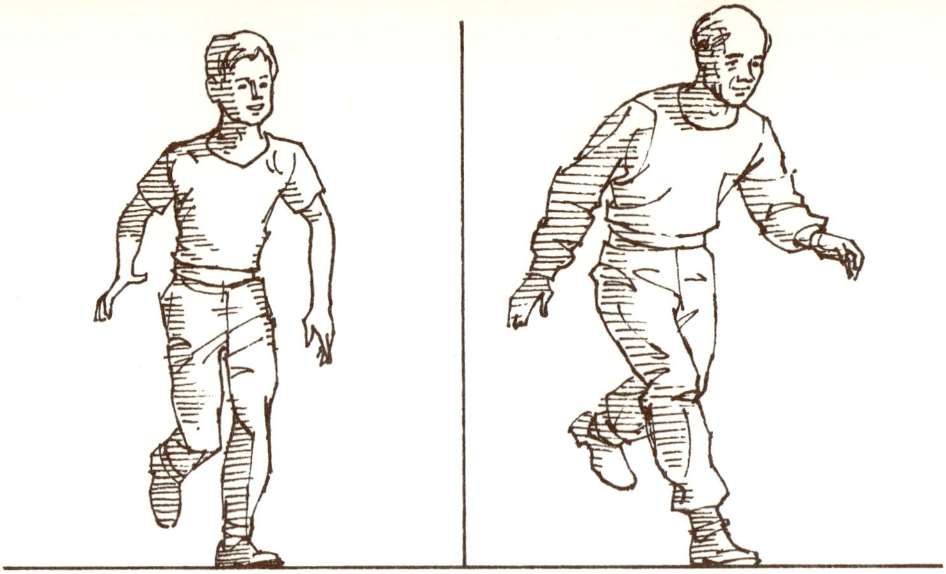

Exercise

Whether a person walks for some special purpose or just for the simple joy of walking, he is getting exercise. Doctors agree that walking is good for the heart and lungs. It keeps muscles, tendons, and ligaments strong and firm. It probably even helps to stimulate some of the thinking functions of the brain. Walking is recommended for lawyers, accountants, secretaries, writers, and others who sit for most of their working day.

Jogging or trotting, alternated with walking, has also become a popular form of exercise. Many Y.M.C.A.'s report that their running tracks are utilized 12 to 15 hours a day. People also run around lakes, around the block, and even in their own homes, where they can jog "in place" by moving their feet up and down rapidly, without going forward.

Jogging is a very easy, convenient, and safe exercise—as well as an effective one—for practically everybody. No special skills or equipment are necessary. A person can run alone or with friends, whenever he chooses. Under medical supervision, jogging is practiced by some elderly people in their 70's and by many people who have weakened hearts.

Even the busiest person can find time to jog. A Massachusetts heart specialist, Dr. Warren R. Guild, usually runs five to eight miles a day, sometimes after midnight. Dr. Guild knows from personal experience that jogging has become an accepted exercise. When the police first saw him running through the streets in the dark of night, they thought something was wrong, and they took him into the station. Now no one pays any attention to him!

Chapter V GAMES, FUN, AND CEREMONY

Most parents remember the very day when a child took his first step. The reason is that the first step showed growth and progress. Most children walk at about 12 or 14 months, but there is no single normal age for starting to walk, and a late walker is just as intelligent as an early walker.

Walking is just the beginning of the ways in which the human foot is used. Stop and think about the actions of your feet, legs, and body when you play. There is hopping, skipping, jumping, leaping, kicking, stamping. You go forward, backward, and sideways, up the monkey bars, down the hill.

Even an ordinary walk can vary. A person does not move the same way on slippery ice as he does on pavement. Have you ever tried to stamp or shake some dirt loose from your shoes while walking? This coordination of mind and muscle differs from the coordination required for the delicate steps you take when someone is sleeping or when you are carrying a very full glass of chocolate milk.

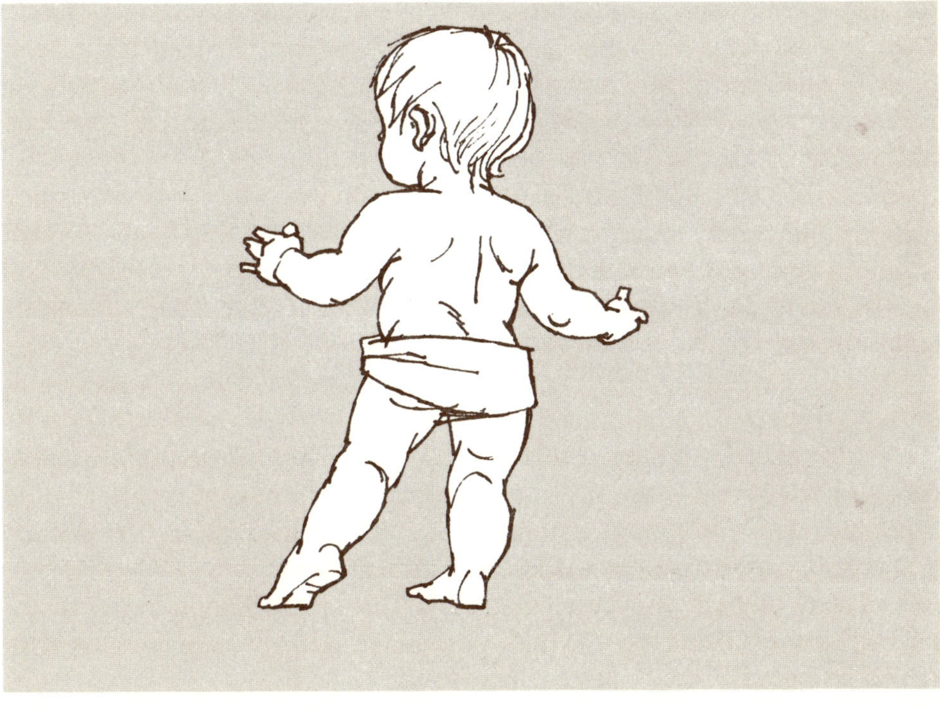

Marches, parades, and processions

Marching is a special kind of walking, when steps are taken in a regular beat or rhythm. Each step covers the same distance as the one before it, and the same number of steps is taken each minute. The United States Army, for example, usually marches in 30-inch steps, at a rate of 120 steps per minute.

To help soldiers stay in step, the commanding officer calls the rhythm or cadence. This is done by shouting numbers in a sing-song fashion . . . one . . . two . . . three . . . four, and then repeating them. The numbers, however, are pronounced more like "hup . . . tup . . . ta-rip . . . foh." On the odd numbers—the "hup" and the "ta-rip". . . the left foot hits the ground. On the even numbers, the right foot hits the ground.

It is fun to watch marchers in parades, which are part of the culture and tradition of practically every country in the world. In the United States, we have parades to celebrate Independence Day and other patriotic holidays, to welcome the New Year and new seasons, to honor heroes, or to advertise a football game or circus. Parades are part of civic festivals, carnivals, and celebrations—the Mardi Gras in New Orleans, the Aquatennial in Minneapolis, the Winter Carnival in St. Paul, Frontier Days in Cheyenne, and the Chinese New Year in Los Angeles and San Francisco. Colorful marching bands make a parade thrilling to hear as well as to see. Almost everyone enjoys rousing march music—the beat of the drum, "oomph" of the tuba, and blast of bugles.

Parades and marches are not always lively. On some occasions, people walk slowly and formally, accompanied by dignified music. These walks are sometimes called processions. You might not ever be in a parade down the middle of your downtown main street, but you almost certainly will be in a procession some day. High school and college graduation exercises generally include a processional march, and so do most weddings.

Processions, parades, and marches can be serious or sad as well as happy. People on demonstration marches carry signs to protest something they think is wrong, or to promote their own cause. When workers go on strike and refuse to work, they set up a procession called a picket line in front of their employer's company. This is intended to be a peaceful way of asking other people not to deal with that company until the strike is settled.

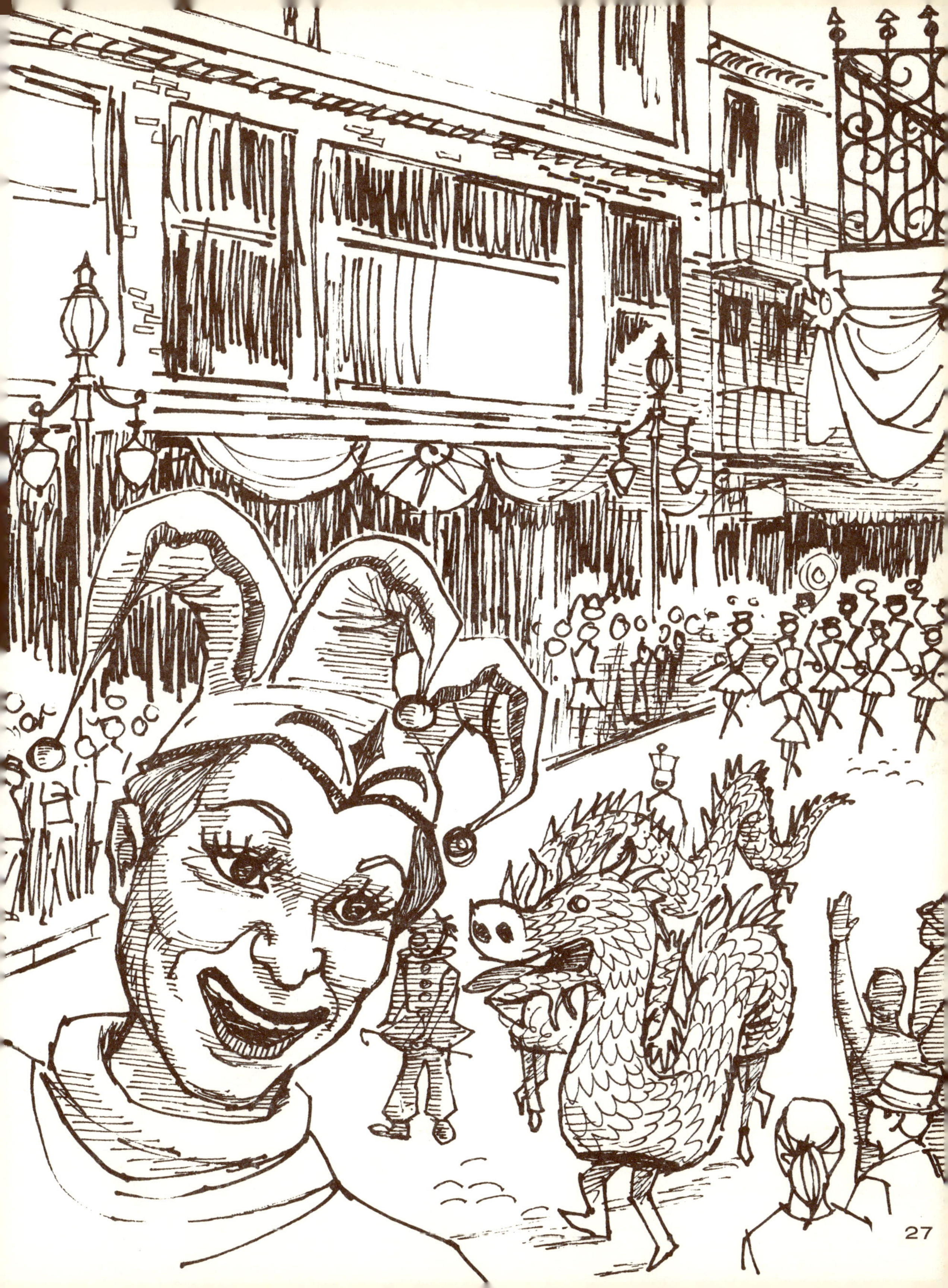

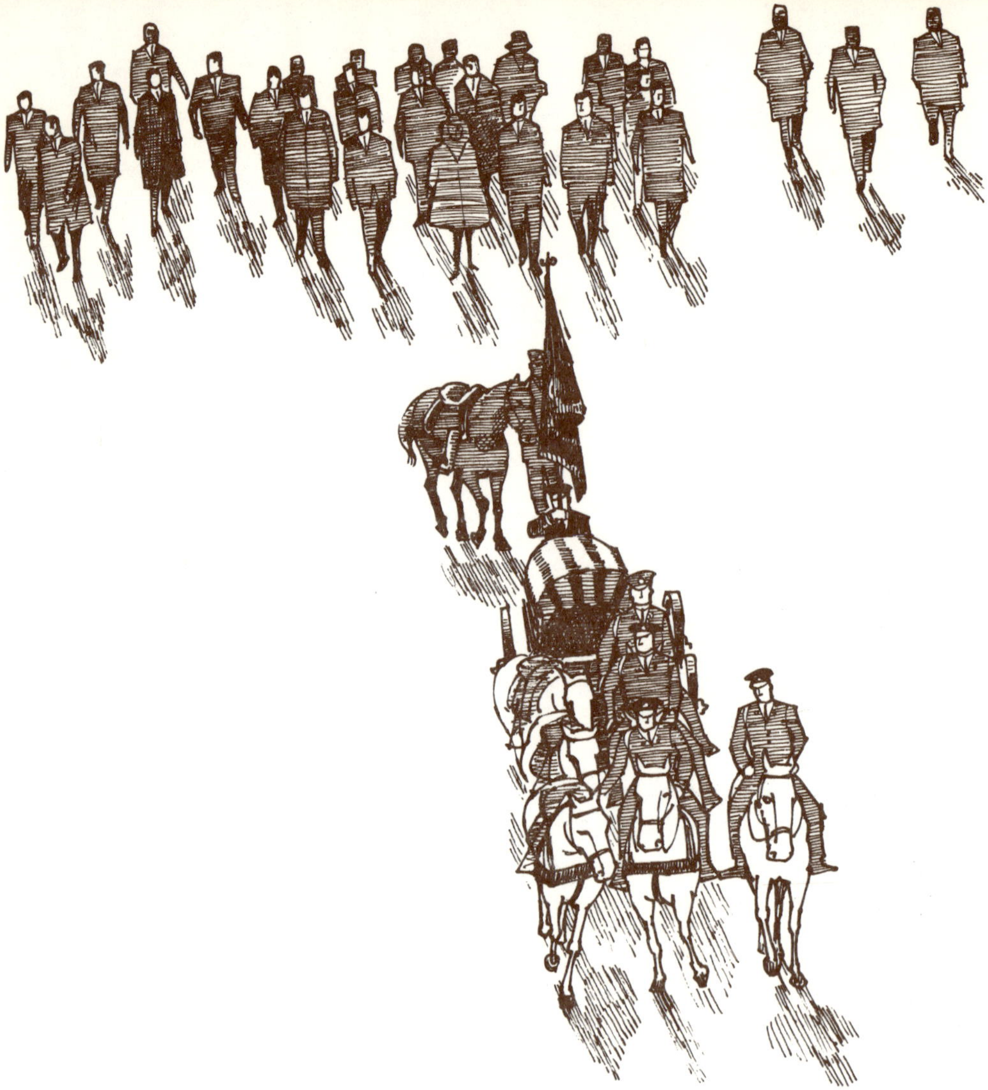

One of the most ancient of processions—and certainly the saddest—is for funerals. Even the caveman probably had a ceremony for carrying the dead to burial grounds. Today in parts of the world where automobiles are not common, people still go on foot to the cemetery.

In this country, during the funeral of President John F. Kennedy on November 25, 1963, the President's widow, Mrs. Jacqueline Kennedy, decided to walk behind the casket in the procession from the Capitol to St. Matthew's Cathedral in Washington, D. C. President Kennedy's brothers, Robert and Edward, walked with Mrs. Kennedy. Behind them, also on foot, were the new President, Lyndon Johnson, and high-ranking officials from almost every country in the world.

Dancing

All uses of the foot—whether the slow pace of the procession, the fast step of the march, or just standing—require balance, coordination, and strength. Some people are stronger and better coordinated than others. But the basic skills can be performed by everyone, except for those with some physical or mental defect.

When more specialized training of foot and body is required, however, we can clearly see differences in ability. Few of us have the balance of gymnasts or ballet dancers. They can remain virtually motionless on one foot while bending so that the body is parallel or horizontal to the floor. Ballet dancers also develop remarkably strong toes, particularly the big toe, since they jump off and land on their toes in many of their movements.

Ballet was first performed in Italy in 1450, and 100 years later appeared in the court of the French King. But dancing itself goes back much farther in history. When early man danced thousands of years ago, before there were any musical instruments, the "music" was supplied by spectators who clapped their hands and stamped their feet.

Primitive dances often had a superstitious purpose; the dancers were trying to cure an illness, or bring rain, or protect men going into battle with the enemy. Later, people danced for sheer pleasure—either their own, or for the enjoyment of their king. They whirled, swirled, leaped high in the air, and bounded across a room like kangaroos. Men and women danced alone and together, and people danced in groups, holding hands. The children's game, "ring around the roses," comes from chain dances given us long ago by the Hebrews and other peoples.

Expert dancers might become professional entertainers, like those who performed in the king's court. We see them today on the stage, in movies, and on television. Their routines are extremely complicated. Each of the thousands of movements is planned by a specialist called a *choreographer,* which means "dance-writer." The choreographer and dancers work together for a long time before a dance is ready to be performed in public.

Sports

In sports, too, the foot is specially trained. Fencers, bullfighters, and boxers depend on rhythm and fast footwork as much as a dancer does. A regular part of a boxer's training program is to skip rope in order to increase his speed-of-foot.

In skiing, skating, and surfing, athletes need strong ankles and durable feet, in addition to an excellent sense of balance and a well-conditioned, well-coordinated body. In football, soccer, and rugby—sports in which a ball is kicked—strong feet and legs are an obvious asset. Some kickers have such tough feet that they can kick a ball barefoot. They use the side of the foot.

The ability to run is important in practically every sport, but in track it is essential. We can guess that early men ran foot races—sometimes in fun, sometimes in earnest. Certainly people on occasion must have had to run for their lives from unfriendly warriors or from dangerous animals.

In 776 B.C., Greece held the first Olympic Games for the greatest runners and throwers in the world. These games, repeated periodically, were among man's outstanding peaceful events until they were halted centuries later by the Roman Empire. The modern Olympic Games were revived by Greece in 1896 and now take place every four years in different cities of the world.

Between Olympics, thousands of track meets are held in the United States and other countries. In every race, from the 100-yard dash to the 26-mile marathon, man is running much more swiftly than he did 10 or 25 or 50 years ago. It used to take 10 seconds for a fast man to run 100 yards. The present record is 9.1 seconds.

Perhaps the most exciting moment for track fans came with the breaking of the "four-minute barrier." For years the greatest milers in the world had attempted to run a mile in under four minutes. Roger Bannister, an Englishman, finally did it, with a time of 3:59.4 on May 6, 1954. Since then, the record has been lowered numerous times. Man will never stop trying to run faster.

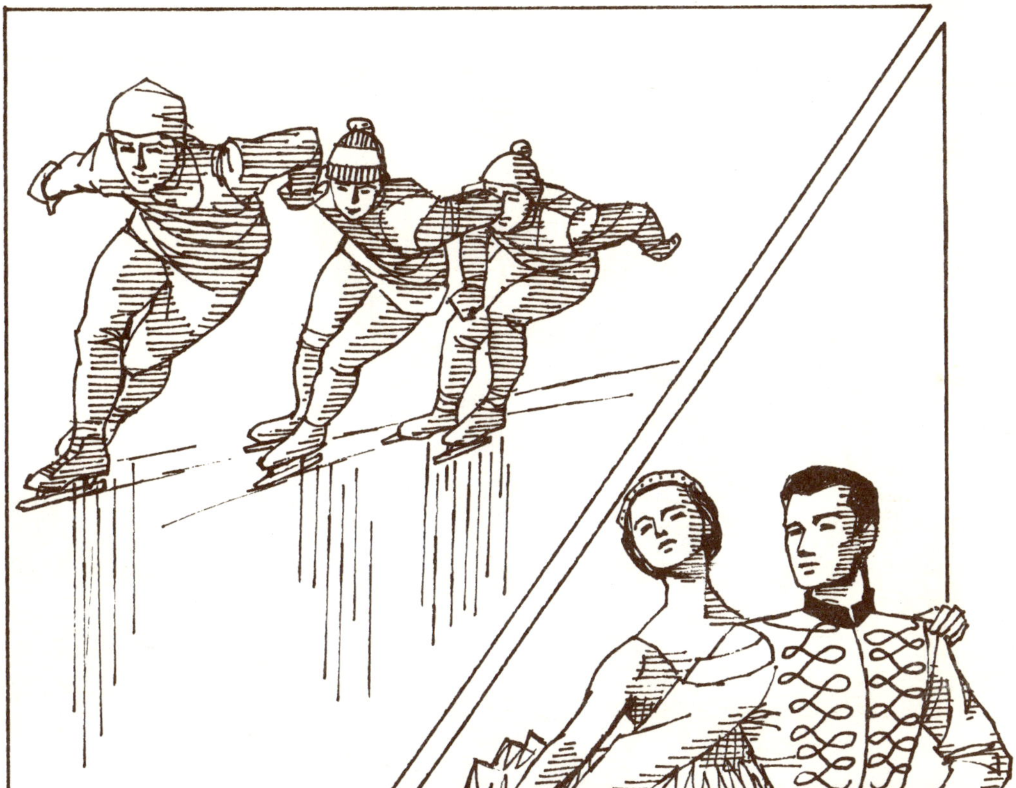

Chapter VI AIDS AND ACCESSORIES

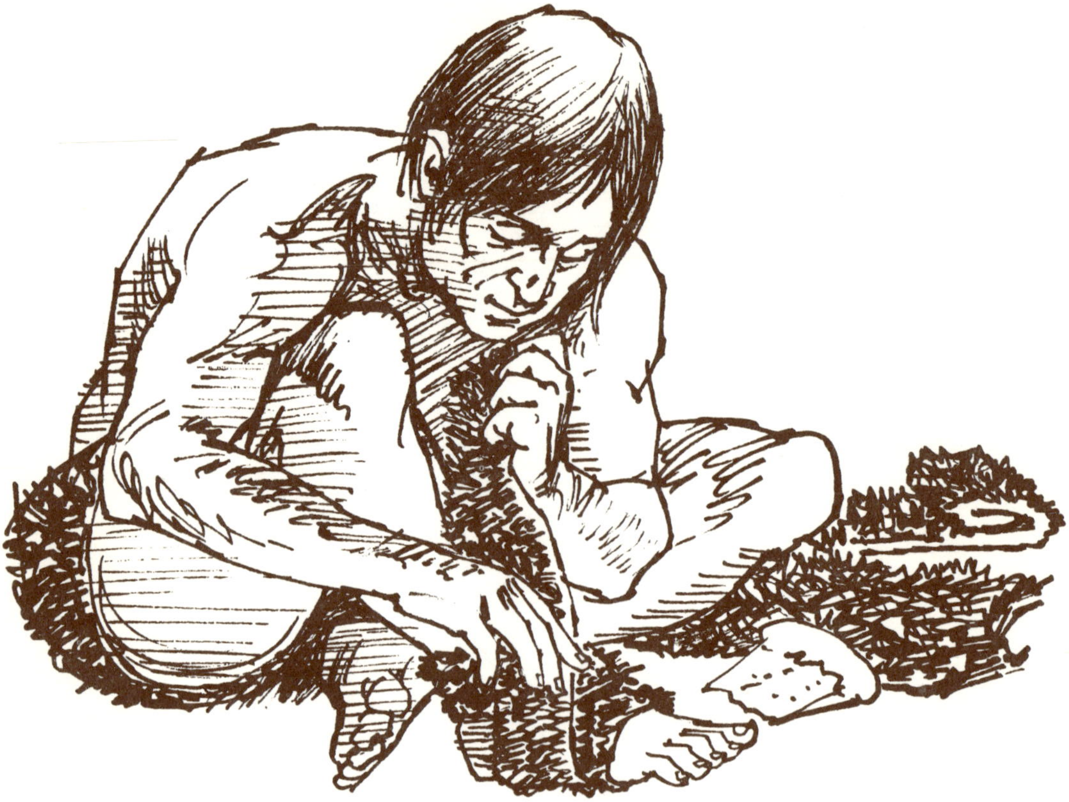

Primitive man made clothing to protect himself from the weather and to shield parts of his body from cuts, scratches, and bruises. He had to devise a special way of protecting his feet, because he depended on them so much. If they got too cold, or too sore, he couldn't hunt for food, or run from his enemies or from dangerous animals. So he trimmed pieces of skin from an animal he had killed, or perhaps he peeled bark from a tree and tied the skin or bark around his feet. These were the first shoes.

The shoe can be considered both an aid and an accessory for the human foot. It is an aid when it protects the foot. It is an accessory when it decorates the foot, or is used for some purpose other than simple protection or support. In the study of footwear, we find that a certain type of shoe might have been an aid at one time and an accessory at another time, depending on who wore it, and why.

Fashions in footwear

In the ancient civilizations of the Near East and the Orient, some people wore shoes with heels in order to keep their feet out of mud, water, snow, or the burning sand of the desert. These heels were a practical aid in walking. But it wasn't long before they were worn for style as well, because women realized that heels improved the appearance of their legs and ankles.

Men wore heels, too. They wanted to be taller. Perhaps they were influenced by actors in Japan, China, and Egypt, who used high heels, and even stilts. This enabled the leading performers to stand out over the other actors on stage.

The height of a heel often indicated a person's wealth or social status. Later, shoes had elevated soles in addition to high heels. In ancient Greece and Rome, some wealthy women had heels and soles so high that they could hardly walk! Other types of footwear, such as sandals, were comfortable as well as luxurious. Colorful and richly decorated, they were worn by both men and women.

One of the customs then was for a new father-in-law to present the bridegroom with an expensive shoe or sandal worn by the bride before her marriage. This symbolized the bride's move from the home of her father to her new home with her husband. The tradition is sometimes carried on today by tying shoes to the automobile of the departing couple.

The look of shoes has changed constantly throughout history. Often one person was responsible for starting a new style for an entire city, or nation. When Catherine de Medici came to Paris in the mid-sixteenth century to marry the future King Henry II, she brought some high heeled shoes with her, starting another wave of popularity for heels.

Men's shoes in the Middle Ages often had long, pointed toes. The beginning of this style goes back to the days of ancient Egypt, when there were slipper-like shoes curving out and up at the toes. About 900 years ago, Fulk Rechin, a noble in the court of England's King William, introduced his own version of the long shoe. He did it for comfort, and to hide the fact that his big toe was swollen. But soon others were wearing pointed shoes too, and each person tried to outdo the other in shoe length. Some footwear was so long and pointed that the ends were tied to the legs with a cord to keep a person from tripping over his own feet.

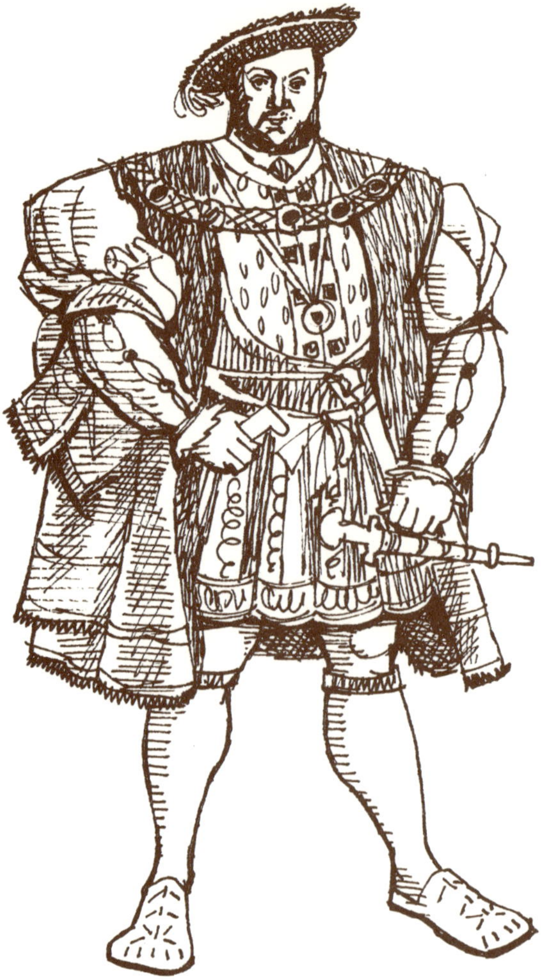

The style changed again in the reign of King Henry VIII, in the early sixteenth century. To ease the pressure on his toes, King Henry needed a shoe which was broad rather than long at the end. When people saw the king wearing broad shoes, they imitated him. Again, each person tried to outdo the other, and eventually some shoes were as wide and silly as those worn today by clowns at a circus.

Another type of footwear, the boot, was designed to cover part of the leg as well as the foot. Generally boots extended to a point just below the knee, although some reached to the thigh and others stopped right at the ankle. Warriors wore boots for protection, as did many people who worked in the fields.

Boots could also be elaborately designed for social occasions. In the early nineteenth century an Englishman named George Bryan Brummell was famous for his fine clothing, including shining black boots. People today still describe a fashionable dresser as a "Beau Brummell." The term is even in the dictionary.

For a very long time, however, footwear was a luxury for most people. They did not have numerous pairs of expensive shoes; they considered themselves fortunate to have one or two pairs of plain shoes, and saved the better pair for holidays or other special events. It was common for stockings to be padded at the bottom so that they could be worn without shoes.

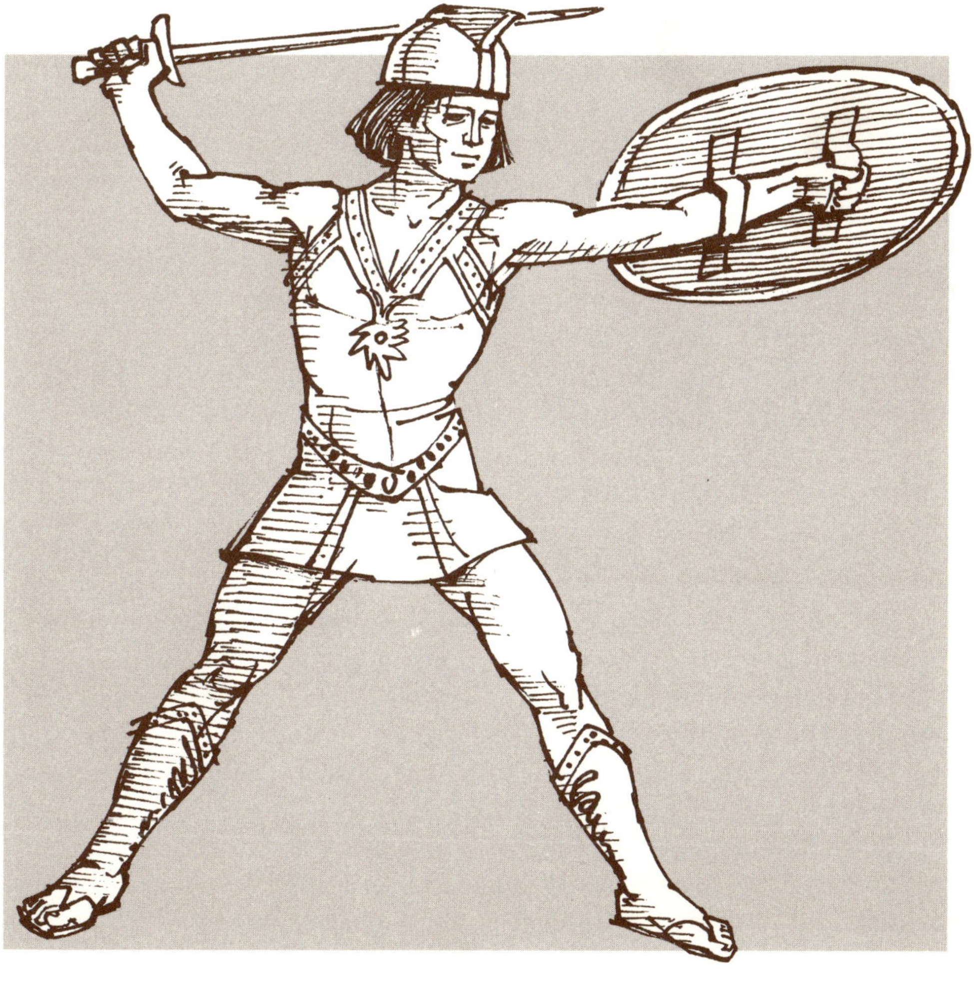

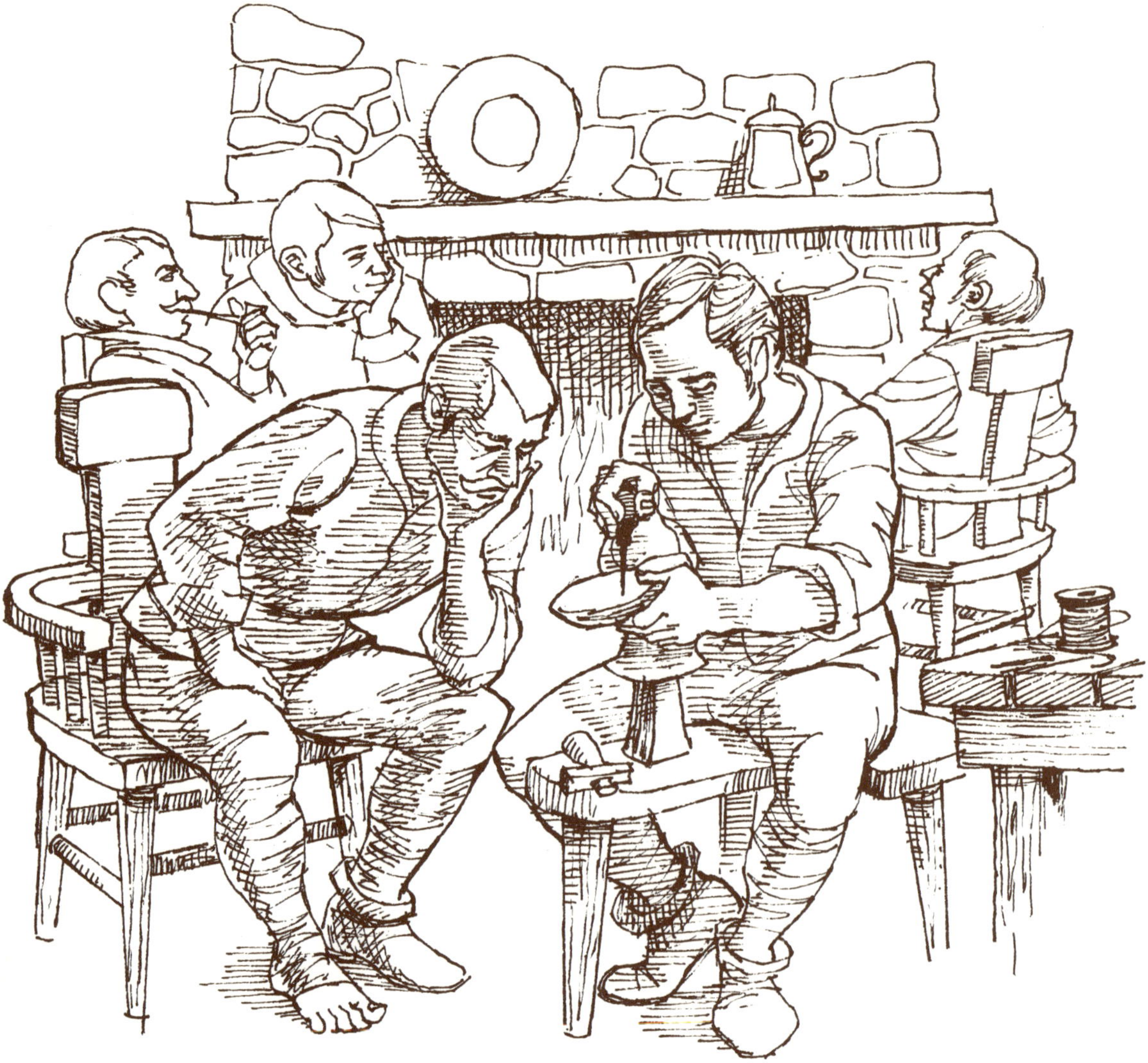

Shoemakers and the shoe industry

The shoemaker was a very important person in most communities. He made shoes as fast as he could—perhaps one pair a day—but he could not keep up with the demand. This was one reason why shoes were a luxury. His shop often was a popular place to meet. Townspeople sat and talked to him while he worked, and chatted among themselves, expressing opinions and trading gossip.

In the English colonies, the first shoemaker was Thomas Beard, who arrived in Salem, Massachusetts in 1629. Soon others followed, setting up shops and teaching the colonists how to make footwear. Much of this instruction took place in Lynn, Massachusetts, which remains to this day one of our country's major shoe manufacturing centers.

Three hundred years ago, shoes were made to fit the feet of the specific customer. The shoemaker measured the length of the customer's foot, guessed at the width, and made a wooden last, or form, to serve as a model for the foot. Then he made the shoes to fit the last. Since there was only one last, the left and right shoes were identical. They could be worn on either foot, and people alternated them to get the most possible use, just as tires are rotated on a car.

In the mid-eighteenth century, shoemakers began making various sizes of shoes to keep in stock. After that, a customer often could find a pair to fit him immediately. But still both shoes were identical. It wasn't until about 100 years later that shoes were designed to fit either the left or the right foot only.

During the past century, numerous changes took place in the shoe industry, as in all industries. Small shops were replaced by huge factories. Sewing machines which could sew leather were developed. Later a machine which cemented the heel to the sole was invented. Today, more than 600 million pairs of shoes are manufactured annually in the United States.

We wouldn't need all of those shoes if we still lived in grassy fields and walked on soft earth. Our feet probably would feel better too, as you have found when you run barefoot through grass or on a sandy beach. There is more "give" and much less pressure from these surfaces than from cement sidewalks, paved streets, and hardwood floors. That's why feet get tired and shoes wear out so fast today.

Fortunately for our feet, the same civilization which makes us walk on hard surfaces also has reduced the number of steps we have to take. We drive downtown in an automobile. In a department store, we do not walk up or down stairs; we take the elevator or escalator. Some day, moving sidewalks will even transport us from one store to another.

Some people say that these developments are bad because we are getting too lazy. Yet the automobile and other methods of transportation are also aids to the feet. A person who enjoys a 10-mile hike through the woods might live 50 miles from the woods. He has to drive to get there. The train and airplane have enabled tourists to visit museums and walk through cities thousands of miles from their homes.

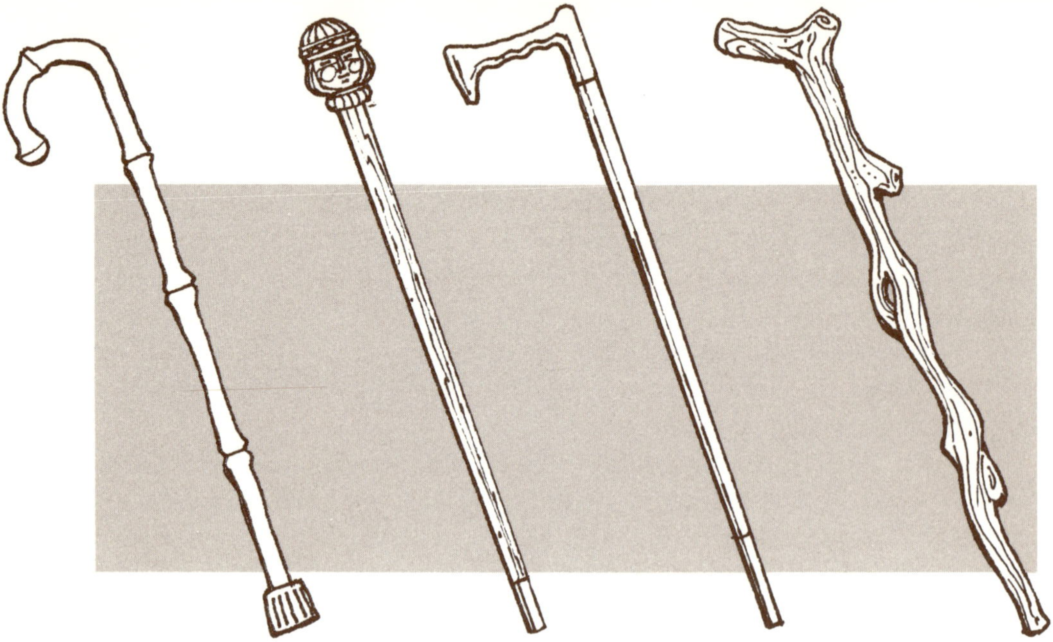

Walking aids

Walking aids must be as old as weapons in the history of man. The heavy stick which was swung at animals also probably served as a support after an injury to the foot. Several hundred years ago, style-conscious men carried expensive, beautifully carved and decorated canes or walking sticks, which were actually fashionable accessories for the hand rather than aids in walking. Today, such accessories are rarely used except as foot supports or as aids to the blind.

When a bone is broken, the foot may require a cast. The cast is a very rigid plaster dressing or wrapping which immobilizes the bones, preventing them from shifting. This allows the break to mend. Casts have been improved over the years. They used to be prepared in the doctor's office, but now they come ready-to-apply. They dry in 15 minutes or so—or about an hour faster—and are several pounds lighter than the early ones.

Sometimes an injury is so severe that a leg or foot must be amputated, or removed. Most amputees, however, can be fitted with an artificial limb made of lightweight wood, metal, or plastic. The sole of the shoe on the limb has a cushion of sponge rubber so that contact with the ground is easier and quieter. It takes time for an amputee to learn to walk with an artificial limb. But his patience is rewarded when he is able to go down the street as naturally as anyone else, attracting no attention whatever.

Chapter VII THE STUDY OF THE FEET

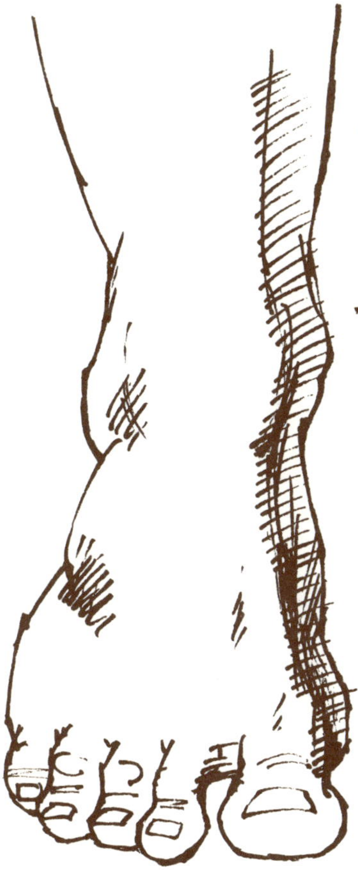

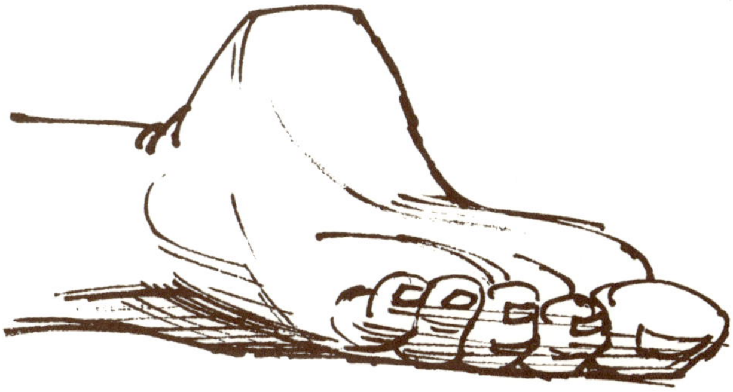

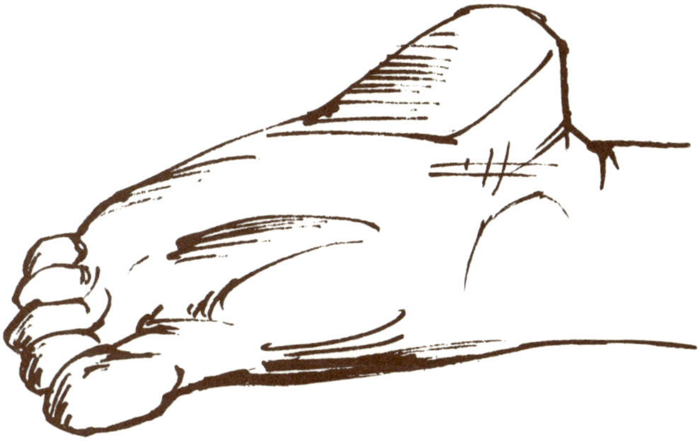

You have probably heard the riddle, "What has a tongue but cannot talk?" The answer, of course, is a shoe. The foot is just the opposite of the shoe. It has no tongue, but it *can* talk.

By talking, we mean that people who study the feet learn things from them, just as you learn from a book, once you understand the words. The foot can tell who we are, how big we are, whether our shoes fit, and even sometimes how healthy we are.

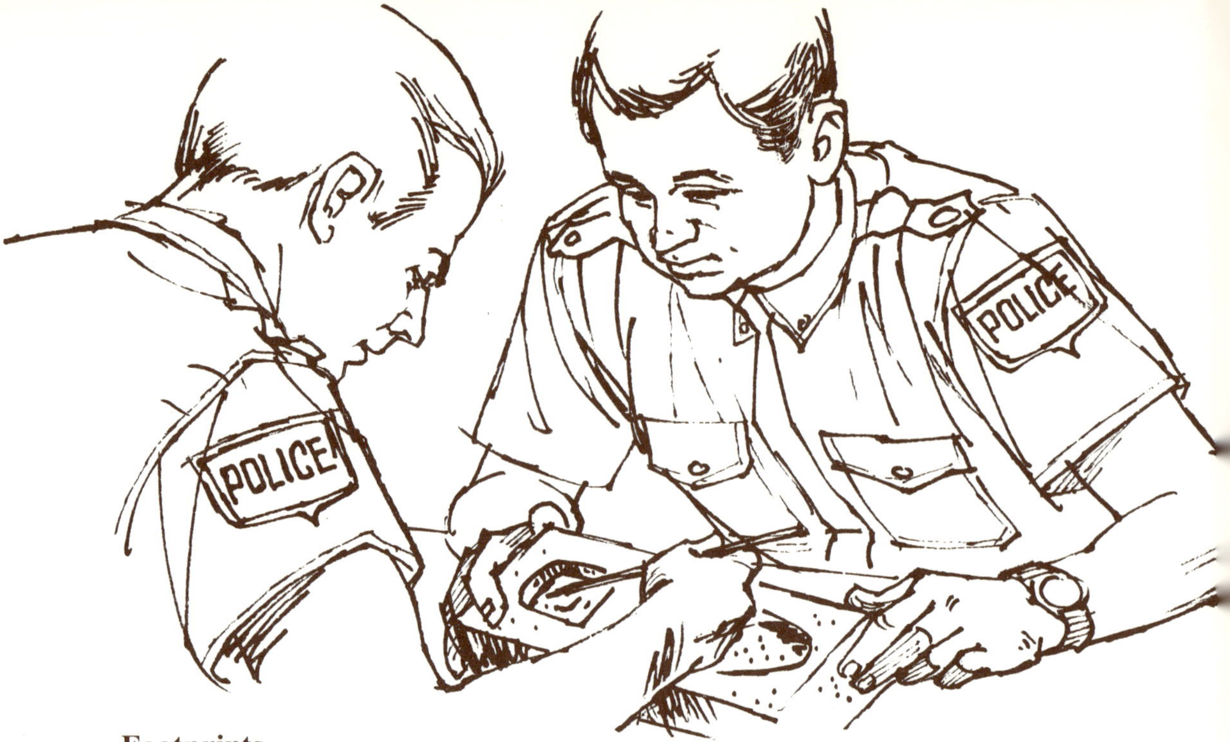

Footprints

Hospital maternity wards, where babies are born, take footprints of the new arrivals. If there is confusion later over which baby belongs to whom, the prints provide positive identification for those trained to read them. No two footprints are alike, just as no two fingerprints are alike.

The prints are made by the many swirling lines, or whorls, in the top or outer layer of skin. This outer layer is called the *epidermis*. Underneath it, and fitting snuggly against it, is another layer of skin known as the *dermis*. The ridges in the dermis form a design of matching ridges and depressions in the epidermis.

Experts in the science of *ichology,* which is the study of tracks, find that impressions made in the ground tell a story as plain as words. They examine clues such as the depth of the heel print, the length of the foot, and the distance between steps. This gives them a very good idea of the height, weight, sex, and age of the individual.

To gain this information, police officers look for tracks after a crime has been committed. Sometimes they are further aided by a distinctive mark from a shoe heel. They can often prove that a person was at the scene of a crime by examining material picked up by his shoes. If it matches material found at the scene, this can be introduced as evidence in court.

Fitting the shoe

When it comes to the study of the foot itself, probably no person — not even a doctor — sees more feet every day than does a shoe salesman. A competent salesman can be very important to the health and comfort of his customers' feet. He is responsible for making sure that shoes fit, although of course there is nothing he can do if a customer insists on the wrong size or style of shoe.

The foot is measured by length and width. The length is indicated by numbers and the width by letters — from AAAA, which is extremely narrow, to EEE, which is very wide. In shoes of the same length, there is a difference of approximately one-sixteenth inch from one width to another. The difference from one full length size to another — 7 to 8, for example — is one-third inch.

A particular shoe size from one manufacturer, however, might differ slightly in actual length or width from that of another manufacturer. Even from the same manufacturer, different styles might vary slightly in actual size, although they have the same number and letter, such as 8B, stamped on the lining. That is why it is best to buy shoes which feel good and fit properly, regardless of the "official" size.

A competent salesman helps the customer find the appropriate shoe. But he never suggests what should be done to the foot itself. The customer should not attempt to treat his foot problems, either. This is a matter which is best left to doctors who, by training and experience, are qualified to deal with problems of the feet.

Foot specialists

Foot specialists fall into two professional categories. One group has the degree, M. D., or Doctor of Medicine. Within this group, doctors who treat the feet are specialists in *orthopedics,* which is the branch of medicine concerned with the bones and joints, including those of the feet. The other foot specialist has the degree, D. P., Doctor of Podiatry, or D. P. M., Doctor of Podiatric Medicine. He receives this degree from one of five recognized Colleges of Podiatry in the United States.

The *podiatrist* used to be called a *chiropodist,* and received a D. S. C. degree, Doctor of Surgical Chiropody. *Chiropody* refers to the treatment of the hand and foot, which originally was the practice of this particular type of doctor. But as chiropodists concentrated increasingly on the foot, they decided it would be more appropriate for them to be known as podiatrists. Podiatry specifically means the treatment or healing of the foot.

The orthopedist and podiatrist are faced with an ever-growing number of minor and major foot problems within the American public. Practically everyone has perfect feet at birth. By the age of 20, however, when the average foot has completed its growth and development, more than seven out of 10 people have had some kind of foot trouble. Among all people, including the elderly, nine out of 10 have had to see a foot specialist sometime during their lives.

Feet may hurt because of ill-fitting shoes or stockings, a breakdown in the structure of the foot, or neglect of foot care. Here are some frequent ailments of the foot:

Athlete's Foot. This is a skin infection with considerable itching and peeling, generally between the toes. Athlete's Foot is not restricted to athletes, although they are more likely to get it than people who never walk barefoot in locker-rooms and gymnasiums.

Bunion. This is an inflammation or swelling which usually occurs between the end of the first metatarsal bone and the big toe. Fulk Rechin, the noble in the court of King William of England, had a bunion. To hide it, he had especially long shoes made.

Corn. Skin thickens whenever and wherever there is continuous rubbing or pressure. Sometimes this is beneficial. African natives, for example, can walk barefoot because of the toughness of the bottoms of their feet. Pressure on toes, however, causes the formation of a thickening, or a corn, which digs *into* the skin and which can be very painful. The corn is one of the most common foot problems.

Fallen Arches. Under severe strain, the bones of the foot—starting with the ankle bone—might slip out of place. The arch then actually sinks or falls, resulting in tired feet and aching legs. Another term for this condition is "flat feet," because the feet indeed become flat. However, flat feet are not necessarily weak. They could simply have a very low arch, which has never broken down and which is as strong as it could be.

Ingrown Toenail. Toenails, like fingernails, are a hardened part of the epidermis protecting blood vessels and sensitive nerve receptors. They are transparent. The pinkish coloring you see is from the blood vessels. Near the bottom or base of the nail, there is less blood circulation and the nail is thicker, giving it a more whitish color. Nails must be

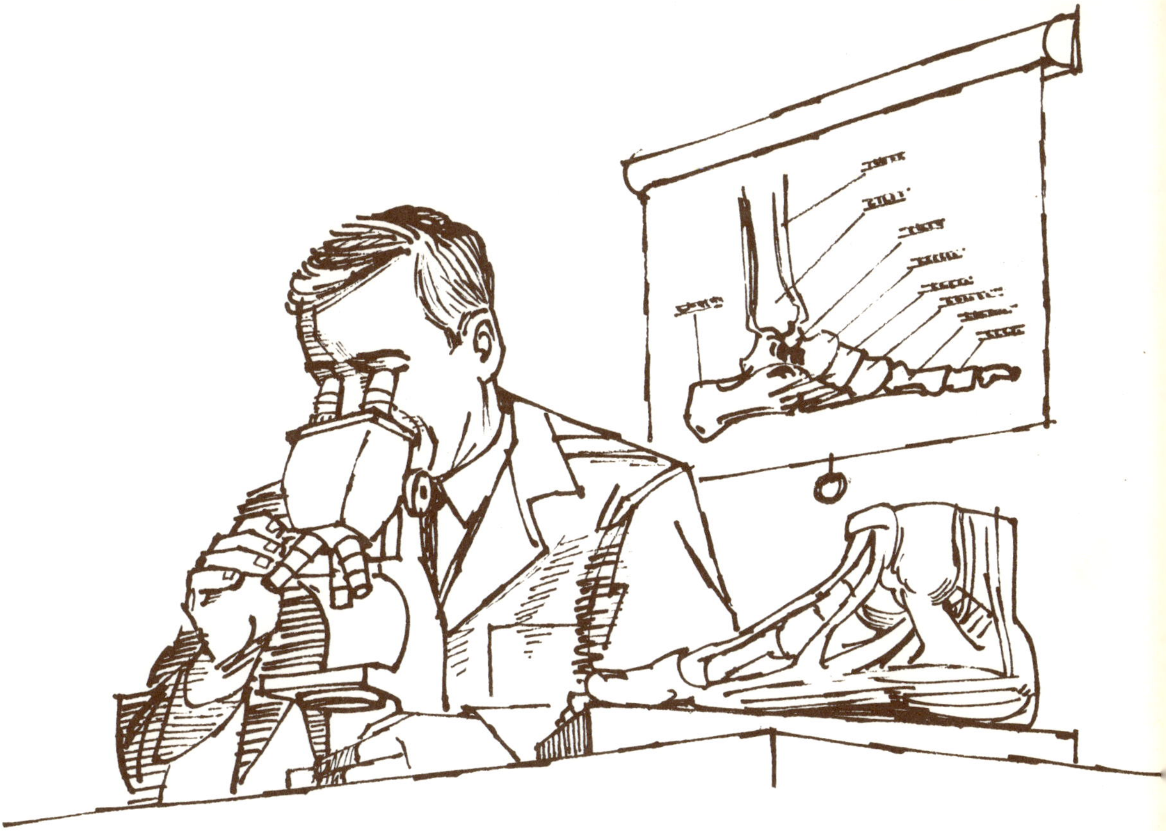

allowed to grow properly. If the shoe or stocking is too short, or if the nail has been carelessly cut or torn away, the edges could start growing into the flesh of the toe.

Doctors are able to aid people with these and many other foot conditions. In addition, an examination of the feet often helps them diagnose general health. Difficulty in walking might be related to problems of the muscles or of balance. Painful feet could be a symptom of arthritis, when there is inadequate lubrication of the joints, or a symptom of diabetes, when the energy-producing sugar of the body is not being sufficiently utilized.

Once the ailment is found, steps can be taken to cure it. Of course doctors do not have all the answers. But new cures and new controls for various diseases are being discovered constantly. People live longer and healthier lives today than they did 100 or 200 years ago, and this progress is expected to continue.

Conclusion THE FUTURE OF THE FOOT

As we move toward the next century, and beyond, what about the future of the foot? Will it continue to serve man as well as it has in the past?

Some people fear that we are getting too lazy, and that our feet and bodies will weaken from too little use. But there are signs that we recognize this danger, and are doing something about it. More people are exercising today than a few years ago. They are listening to doctors and others who say, "Go for a walk."

In business and industry, some modern planners even suggest offices with "stand-up" desks and other arrangements which will prevent employees from sitting practically all day. Research indicates that a person is more alert if he moves around.

There will always be some foot problems. But problems do not make the foot any less remarkable. Just look at how much the feet can do *in spite* of the fact that they often hurt! Let's go one step further – think of how much the feet could do if they *didn't* hurt! Fortunately, people *can* have healthier feet in the future. Orthopedists and podiatrists can cure most of the common ailments, if they get the chance soon enough.

Learn how to take care of your remarkable feet. Appreciate them, and they will serve you well.

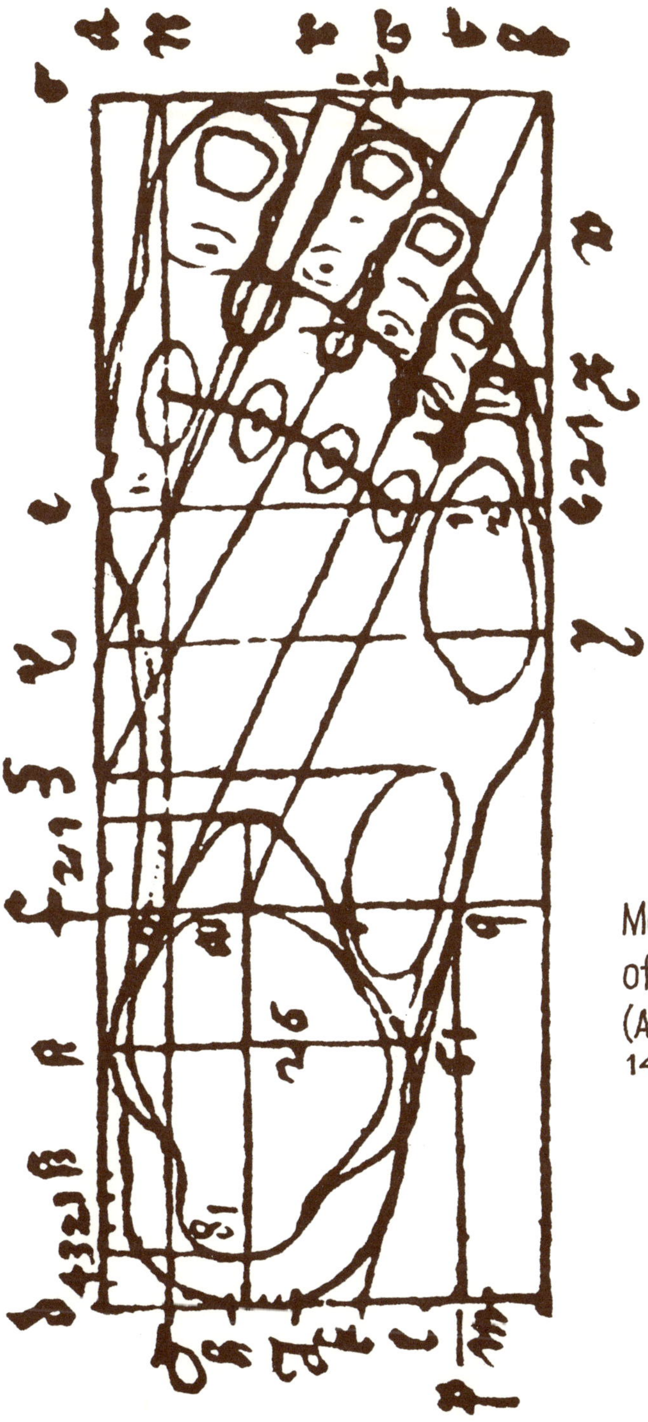

Measurements of the Foot (Albrecht Dürer 1471-1528)

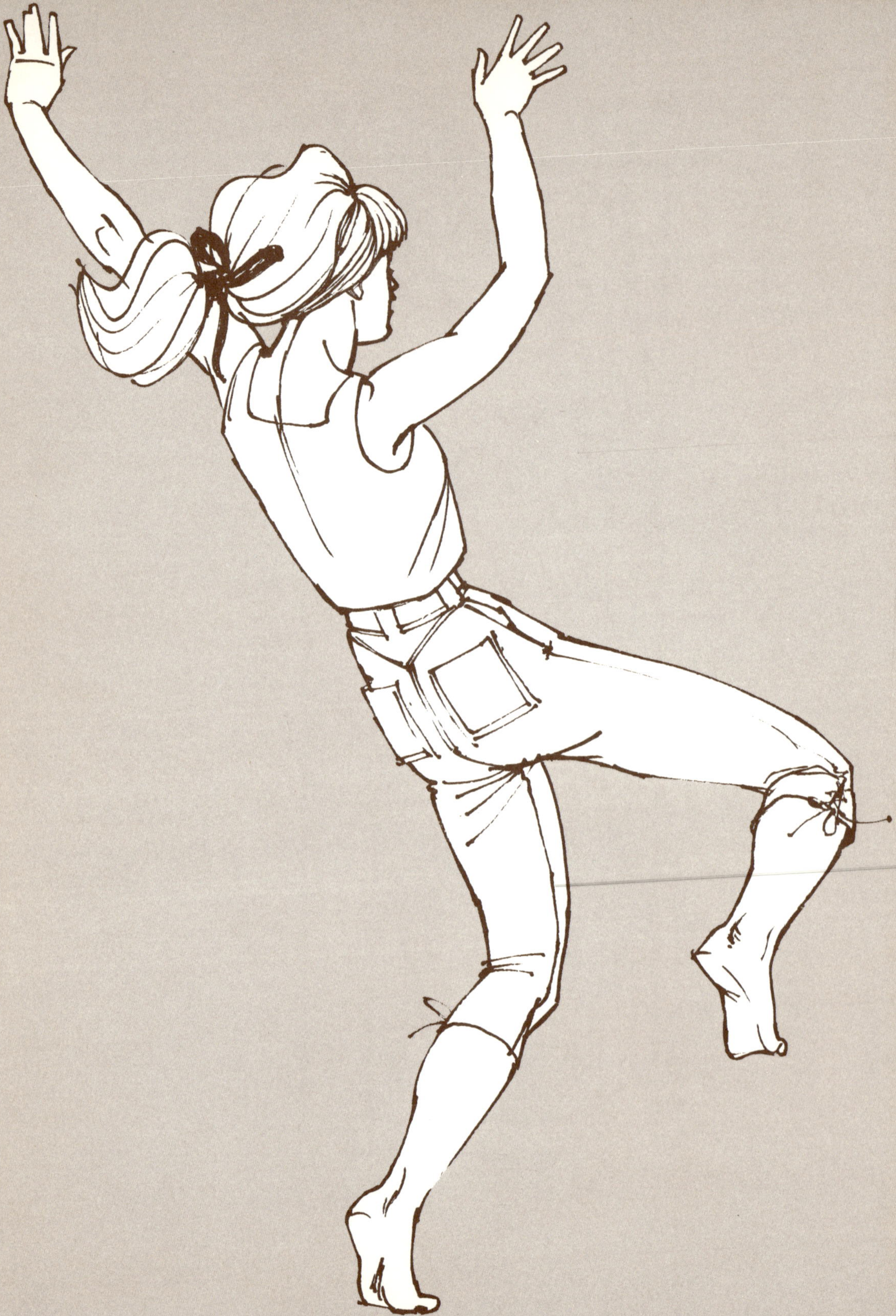

Robert K. Krishef

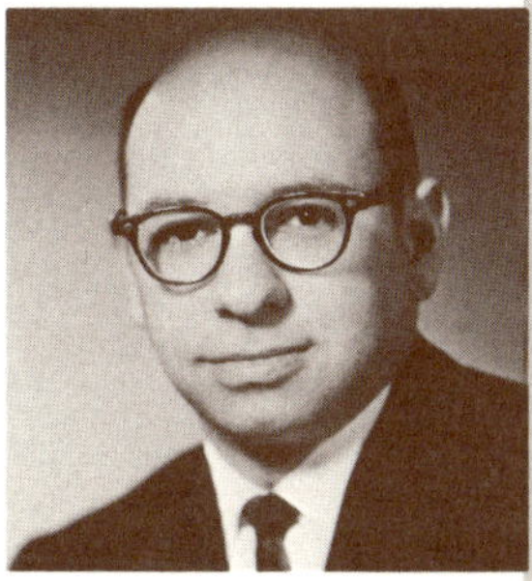

Robert K. Krishef recalls writing his first short story "when I was about 10 years old." He has been involved in writing, in one form or another, ever since. Krishef, who was born and raised in Minneapolis, holds Bachelor's and Master's degrees in Journalism from the University of Minnesota. An experienced ex-newspaperman and later a free lance writer, he has been a reporter, sports editor, and city editor on daily and weekly newspapers, and has written fiction and articles for various magazines. Presently he is director of public relations with an advertising agency. He resides with his wife and their two children in St. Louis Park, a suburb of Minneapolis.

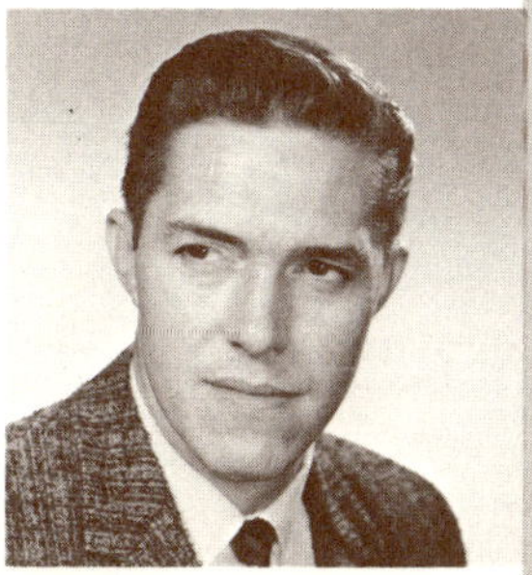

Harold K. Lamson

Harold K. Lamson is an experienced artist and illustrator. Born and raised in Wisconsin, Lamson served in the United States Army during World War II. He then attended River Falls State Teachers College, the University of Minnesota, and the Minneapolis School of Art where he graduated with honors. Since then his work has appeared in many important exhibits, and in 1956 he won the "Best of the Show" award at the Minnesota State Fair Exhibit. Lamson and his family reside in Minneapolis.